AYAHUASCA
MEDICINE

"Alan Shoemaker has seen it all, and done it all. In this book he narrates his life story with humor and passion. A read sure to be of interest!"

DENNIS MCKENNA, PH.D., ETHNOPHARMACOLOGIST
AND AUTHOR OF *BROTHERHOOD OF THE SCREAMING ABYSS*
AND COAUTHOR OF *THE INVISIBLE LANDSCAPE*

"Ayahuasca Medicine is a revealing journey on the Western shamanic path with one of the most preeminent gringos on the Iquitos frontier. Alan Shoemaker's apprenticeship with the medicine ayahuasca is rich in wonder, frank in detail, and embodies the cultural metamorphosis those of us who connect with the power plants must undergo. And as a new generation of Western seekers comes to the jungle in search of the mystery, Alan's greatest wisdom may be his understanding that true healing comes from within. As well as the plants and the curanderos, Westerners are being groomed to be their own teachers, and Alan Shoemaker stands foremost among them."

RAK RAZAM, AUTHOR OF
AYA AWAKENING: A SHAMANIC ODYSSEY

AYAHUASCA
MEDICINE

The Shamanic World of
Amazonian Sacred Plant Healing

ALAN SHOEMAKER

Park Street Press
Rochester, Vermont • Toronto, Canada

Park Street Press
One Park Street
Rochester, Vermont 05767
www.ParkStPress.com

Park Street Press is a division of Inner Traditions International

Library of Congress Cataloging-in-Publication Data
Shoemaker, Alan.
  Ayahuasca medicine : the shamanic world of amazonian sacred plant healing /
Alan Shoemaker.
      pages cm
  Includes index.
  Summary: "An insider's account of the journey to become an ayahuasquero, a
shaman who heals with the visionary vine ayahuasca" — Provided by publisher.
  ISBN 978-1-62055-193-6 (pbk.) — ISBN 978-1-62055-194-3 (e-book)
  1. Shamanism. 2. Ayahuasca ceremony. 3. Hallucinogenic plants. 4.
Hallucinogenic drugs and religious experience. I. Title.
  GN475.9.S56 2014
  299.8'131—dc23
                                                              2013023539

Printed and bound in the United States by Versa Press

10 9 8 7 6 5 4 3 2 1

Text design and layout by Brian Boynton
This book was typeset in Garamond Premier Pro with Omni and Gill Sans as
display typefaces

To send correspondence to the author of this book, mail a first-class letter to the
author c/o Inner Traditions • Bear & Company, One Park Street, Rochester, VT
05767, and we will forward the communication, or contact the author directly at
alanshoemaker@hotmail.com.

For my children, Liam and Claire Shoemaker,
and to the spirits of the plants

CONTENTS

Foreword by Peter Gorman   ix

Introduction   1

                     ⁎

The Quest   4

Synchronicities   7

Dr. Valentin Hampjes   11

San Pedro   18

Breaking through Barriers   28

In Search of a Maestro   34

Return to Ecuador   47

Don Jose Fatima   61

Don Fernando's Brew   65

The Power of the Icaros   75

Don Juan Tangoa, Ayahuasquero   80

The Spirit World   95

Diet   102

My Initiation   105

Epilogue   115

※

Appendix 1. No Shortcuts   120

Appendix 2. The Price of Learning   123

Appendix 3. Two Icaros from Don Pedro   126

Glossary   129

About the Author   136

Index   137

FOREWORD

BY PETER GORMAN

Alan Shoemaker first arrived in Iquitos, Peru, in 1993, and he arrived with a bang, coming down the Putumayo with several friends in a fifteen-meter-long dugout canoe with a forty-horsepower Yamaha motor. He'd come from Washington State via Ecuador, where he had studied with Dr. Valentin Hampjes, the noted medical doctor and curandero/shaman who was as familiar with San Pedro cactus and ayahuasca as he was with antibiotics.

I didn't intend to spend a lot of time thinking about Alan Shoemaker when he first arrived in Iquitos. I'd been using this water-bound city for nine years as a staging point for my work in the jungle before he'd ever set foot there. I'd already met two dozen Shoemakers who always showed up in town, thought it was an easy place to get by, and then discovered, three months later, that they were calling family and friends for money to get home. But this gringo turned out to be different from most of the other dreamers I'd met. It turned out, as Alan later explained to me, that while wondering where to go for a break from his teacher, Valentin, he'd picked up a copy of *Shaman's Drum,* a wonderful magazine produced by Timothy White that deals with all things shamanistic. This particular issue included an article on ayahuasca written by me. And that led Alan to Iquitos, my haunt.

Now, for better or worse, I'd written the first nationally published article about ayahuasca, for *High Times* magazine, in 1986. Yes, Burroughs and Ginsberg had written about it previously in *The Yage Letters,* published in 1963 by San Francisco–based City Lights, but that collection of correspondence and other writings had not quite captured national attention like my article did more than twenty years later. My piece on ayahuasca resounded in those pre-Internet times and was passed around from person to person, until probably more than a million people had read it. As a result, several thousand people decided to seek out the medicine.

The article Alan had read still had influence. And so he showed up at my second home. But that is an understatement. He showed up, and within a month or two he launched the first modern English-language newspaper in Iquitos. A few months after that, he was making large batches of ayahuasca in the street in front of his residence—to the delight of the locals.

He worked with several curanderos, but seemed to focus on Juan Tangoa, whom we affectionately called Airport Juan, because his home is on a block in a barrio very close to the Iquitos airport. But Alan didn't just work with Don Juan: he became the first gringo to take a Peruvian curandero on a public tour of the United States and Europe. And while others might have done that previously, Alan did it with flair, introducing the concept of the traveling curandero to the world.

As with that particular tour, everything else Alan did, he did with great flair. Certainly everything you might know about Iquitos and ayahuasca has been influenced—some say for better, others say for worse, but still, the influence is not disputed—by Alan. Within a couple of years of landing in Iquitos, Alan set up a small souvenir shop just off what is now "the boulevard." Not long afterward a young woman came to town looking to drink ayahuasca. She wound up going with Alan to drink the medicine with Francisco Montes, at a place Don Francisco's family had bought him out on the then-uncompleted road to Nauta, at kilometer 18. The young woman had such a transformative experience that she tried to give Alan a $500 bonus for his work, but Alan refused, suggesting instead that she give the money to Don "Poncho" Francisco as seed money to create the first ethnobotanical garden in Iquitos, starting with identifying and marking all the medicinal plants on his property. She did so, and from that first $500, Sachamama Ethnobotanical Garden, the first ayahuasca center, was born in 1990. Every other center that has been founded since then owes a debt of gratitude not only to Sachamama, but to Alan as well.

For me, the first hint that something extraordinary was happening occurred around 1995. During the late 1980s, whenever I flew into Iquitos from Miami on the now-defunct Faucett Airlines, there were always two, three, or four wheelchair-bound end-stage AIDS patients aboard. When we reached Iquitos they were whisked off the plane and into cars, quickly disappearing into the night. After perhaps the third time I observed this, my curiosity was so piqued that I managed to slip off the plane with a group of them, got a taxi, and followed them. They wound up at the river's edge and were loaded onto a fairly small boat, which took off and disappeared from view.

Something was up. These were end-stage patients. There was no going home unless there was a miracle. So I began asking around town about them. I got word here and there about some strange, near-blind bear of a doctor who was doing experimental work on them, but I could never pin it down. I just could not find out what was what, though I knew that something was up. Then around 1995, when I came down to Iquitos for a few months, Alan told me he had taken what I'd said and had actually located the doctor doing the work with the AIDS patients. His name was Dr. Roberto Inchaustegui, and he was treating those dying people with a mixture of an Upper Amazonian medicinal plant and other things. And while most of those people still died, some survived, and a few even thrived. It was Alan who had found the doctor I could not find.

A year or so later it was Alan who introduced me to the idea of ayahuasca healing in a way I'd never considered. Remember, there were a few books on the subject, but the Internet did not exist then so there was no way of doing research—just the experiential knowledge of a few who had taken the medicine. Alan came to me one day and told me his mother was dying and asked me to drink ayahuasca with him at Airport Juan's house to see if we might not see what was killing his mom and what might help her to stay alive. I reluctantly agreed, sure I could not help.

That night, during the ceremony, I saw her issue, up close and personal, and saw that uña de gato would help her. I wrote a note when I saw that, and the next morning I showed my note to Alan, sure that I was crazy. Alan had written a note as well, which also said "uña de gato," as well as "jergón sacha." He sent or brought the medicines to his mom—I forget which—and some months later, his mother, who was supposed to die within weeks, was told by her doctors that they could not find any cancer, and that they might have misdiagnosed her to begin with. Alan and I knew better.

Several years later Alan came with me and my mother-in-law, Lydia, a Peruvian woman two generations out of jungle tribal life, to Airport Juan's to help heal Lydia's cancer. It worked. She got several more good years, just like Alan's mom did.

Alan's biggest drawback was that he loved being the tallest rose in the garden. And he often was. He was the first gringo to set up an official plant export company in Iquitos. Large companies had done it earlier, but no one had done it on a personal level like Alan did. To do it, he had to learn how Peruvian corporations were set up, what papers and permits were needed, and how to satisfy both U.S. and United Nations bureaucracies. It took years of painstaking work. It was done in part with the help of my family's "paper man," Jorge

"Flaco" Panduro Perea, the best man at moving paper in all of Iquitos. He never missed or misses a trick. He set up Alan and his then-wife, Mariella, as a unique company capable of moving plant material legally from Peru to anywhere in the world.

Life, somehow, seems to intervene at the most awkward moments. I had a bar in Iquitos, the Cold Beer Blues Bar, across the street from the Puerto Mastranza, on the toughest block in town. Tourists were terrified of going there; my clients included expatriates, locals, U.S. Special Forces, and every CIA/DEA/NSA personnel in Iquitos at any given time—that and every drug dealer, arms dealer, and any other person the CIA/DEA/NSA was interested in. Well, as luck would have it, some of those young bucks from the United States would get drunk and cry into their beers to the bartender—who was often me. Now, everybody knew I was a journalist, and I told everybody that whatever they told me at the bar was likely to be published if I thought it newsworthy, so we didn't do any sneak attacks. Still, over the course of the couple of years I had the bar, at least two or three black ops were stopped in their tracks when I published stories about them on Al Giordano's seminal NarcoNews.com website.

And, as luck would have it, a couple of former Navy Seals who were working for the CIA as mercenaries were at my bar one night, at a party we were having for some guests I was taking to the jungle. Well, one of the guests took a photo of me behind the bar. One of the ex-Seals thought she might have captured his image via the mirrors behind the bar, so he walked over to her, ripped her camera from her neck, and stepped on it, breaking it. His lieutenant called him on the infraction, and the drunk mercenary then ate a bar glass. That's right, simply ate an entire six ounces of glass, out of shame. But before he did that he told me what he and the other former Seals were in town to do: they were planning to head up the Putumayo River to slaughter any and all persons trying to escape a pincer movement planned by U.S. and U.S.-trained Colombian forces for the following month.

There would be bonuses of $1,000 for every confirmed kill, whether combatant or civilian man, woman, or child, he said.

I wrote up the story and the op was canceled.

A couple of days later I was in my friend Jim's Gringo Bar. At one table was the lieutenant with a local girl. I sat with them while Alan stayed at the bar. The fellow told me I was in serious trouble for mucking up the operation. I told him I respected the military, but not the idea of trying to force civilians to flee a U.S.-paid onslaught on the Colombian rebels in a thirty-year-old civil war that would result in him and his fellows making money on killing fleeing civilians. Then, for some reason that seemed to make sense to me at the time, I decided to "soplar," the fellow. *Soplar*, is a blessing wherein you take magic liquid into your mouth and spray a fine mist over someone's head and body to cleanse their aura. I didn't have any sacred liquid, so I used beer. The lieutenant didn't see it as a blessing—he thought I had spit at him, and in an instant he had his finger around my thorax and told me he might kill me. I told Alan to explain that I was blessing him to not kill noncombatants, not spitting at him. Alan, the tallest rose in the garden, seized the moment and hurled a hailstorm of shit on the fellow's head, making it clear that not only was his position finished, but that he would likely wind up doing hard time for attacking a journalist such as Peter Gorman.

The fellow took it seriously. He let go of me but told Alan that he would pay for the incident.

And pay he did. A few months later, Alan, with all the proper paperwork in the world, sent a huge shipment of *Banisteriopsis caapi*—ayahuasca vine, maybe 700 pounds of it—along with chacruna (*Psychotria viridis*) and chaliponga (*Diplopterys cabrerana*, also known as huambisa after the tribe of the same name) the admixture plants used to make ayahuasca, the black tobacco (*Nicotiana rustica,* known also as mapacho) native to Peru, and some other things to the Atlanta address of his ex-wife, who was an attorney for the EPA, for delivery to his son. Now, what Alan did was perfectly legal. And if U.S. Customs had not wanted to receive the shipment they had two options: they could say the plant material was not wanted in the United States, and they could either destroy it or return it to the sender on the sender's dime. Of course, if the material had been mislabeled it would have been smuggling. But as all the material was labeled properly in both English and Spanish, with local and Latin names, that was not the case. Nonetheless, U.S. Customs permitted the shipment to go through . . . and then arrested Alan's grown son for picking it up off his front lawn.

Despite this outlandishly illegal move by the U.S. Attorney's office, which it turned out was instigated by the former Seal lieutenant who said to "get Shoemaker and Gorman" (a fact that was stated to me on the record by the DEA), when Alan tried to go through Atlanta to get to his mother's bedside just before her death he was picked up, put on a bus, and delivered to prison for thirty days. His mother died two days after his arrest. Thereafter Alan was given house arrest and was not permitted to leave the States or even go farther than a block or two from the home of his deceased mom. That lasted just under one year, the limit the U.S. federal prosecutors had to either prosecute him for a crime or let him go. Well, they had no crime to prosecute him for; the only crime committed was done by U.S. Customs in allowing legal plants to go through and then arresting Alan and his son.

So after 360 days, and I might be off by one or two, but just shy of the limit, the U.S. Attorney returned Alan's suitcase, which contained his passport. Alan was originally arrested on April 1st. One year to the day later he received a letter stating he no longer had travel restrictions and so was free to leave the country. Alan came to my home in Texas, where he stayed for a couple of weeks, overseeing a study run by a doctor to determine if the medicinal plants he had been successfully using in Iquitos to put high blood sugar into remission would stand up to the rigors of a formal test. During that time I called the judge, a U.S. attorney, and everyone else and got it confirmed that Alan was free to travel, so long as he'd be available should they ever decide to prosecute. At that point, Alan, who had not seen his wife or kids for a year, bought a ticket to Lima and on to Iquitos. I double-checked with the judge and prosecutor. And finally, knowing I had everyone on tape saying he could leave, I drove my friend to the Dallas/Fort Worth Airport and sent him on his way.

Less than a week later the prosecuting attorney in Atlanta charged Alan with flight to avoid prosecution—a ridiculous lie considering she was on tape suggesting he should visit his wife in Peru. Unfortunately for Alan, if he ever returns to the States he'll have to answer to that charge before any ayahuasca charges can be addressed—which means that unless he's got a quarter of a million dollars in legal fees put away, he's sunk.

But none of that sunk him.

He went back to Iquitos to discover that his family had had a hard time without him. He countered by coming up with the idea of a shamanistic conference. He brought in some inspiring speakers, collected several good curanderos to offer medicine to the participants, and began what has now become an annual event. And out of those conferences, the thriving business of ayahuasca tourism in Iquitos and Pucallpa was born.

So Alan's fingerprints, more than anyone else's, have been on all things ayahuasca in Iquitos. Even the beautiful *mantas,* or weavings, done by the indigenous Shipibo that are sold in Iquitos and Pucallpa bear his influence: at the very first shaman conference the weavers incorporated the Vine of the Soul (Soga del Alma) logo, a stylized cross section of an ayahuasca vine—imagined by Alan and later drawn by Johan Fremin—into their weavings, and now depictions of ayahuasca appear on nearly all of the mantas the Shipibo sell. The Bora tribe is now also painting his logo as well.

Alan is loved by many. He's also been called every name in the book, by people of all stripes. But few of those people have ever walked a mile in his shoes. Few of those people have had the courage he has shown. I am not always his biggest fan. I wish he had not set Sachamama and all of the subsequent ayahuasca retreats in motion. I wish it could all have been kept secret and slowly let out over the next fifty years, rather than just taking it to the streets. But that doesn't mean I am right. History will tell.

What needs to be known is this: That he's my brother—good, bad, or in-between. And I fight for his right to be the tallest rose in the garden.

Enjoy his story. Enjoy this book.

PETER GORMAN is an award-winning investigative journalist who has spent more than twenty-five years tracking down stories, from the streets of Manhattan, to the slums of Bombay, to the jungles of Peru. Gorman worked for *High Times* magazine for fourteen years as a senior editor, executive editor, and as editor-in-chief. His feature writing and editorials have appeared in dozens of major national and international magazines, he has consulted for both National Geographic's *Explorer* series and the BBC's *Natural World,* and he has appeared in several documentaries and hundreds of radio programs. He is the author of *Ayahuasca in My Blood: 25 Years of Medicine Dreaming.*

INTRODUCTION

Shamanic healing has been around for thousands of years and will remain for thousands more. During the Eurocentric age of reason, the birth of empiricism and materialism, we were led away from believing in things we could not see and hear, that we could not place in our hands and feel and weigh. This contrived reality found its way to the Americas a little over 500 years ago, and through force of arms, unknown viruses, and the Spanish Inquisition, it ravaged cultures and humiliated the medicine men, taking away their gods and forcing them into submission. There remained, however, a few daring souls who continued to practice their magic, hidden from the death threats of the conquistadors.

At the National University of Peru in Iquitos can be found a scientist hard at work in his test tube–laden lab, processing one of the Sacred Power Plants, ayahuasca, into powdered form. Ayahuasca is an *entheogen,* meaning "generating the Divine within"; it is a medicinal plant that has been used for thousands of years by Amazonian shamans (see appendix 1). For years this scientist has been busy trying to decipher the secrets of this ancient medicine, with few new insights. The efforts to determine the alkaloid constituents that produce ayahuasca's celebrated visions and hallucinations were easily accomplished, but, says the scientist, "We still cannot figure out how a group of five people all drinking the same ayahuasca at the same time can have the

1

same hallucination at the same moment." Such is the pity in being a scientist.

"What you are trying to measure or weigh cannot be done," I told him. "Whatever intricacies of this medicine you are trying to intellectually discover will always leave you one short. No matter what you do, how many tests you make, or how numerous the compounds you find, your scientific method will never get you to the bottom of this mystery. Why? Because you cannot measure God, you cannot weigh the Divine."

"Yes, I know that," he replied. "But I am a scientist. This is what I must search for, what I have to do."

What a thankless task, looking for the Light in a test tube! How do you factor the Divine in a scientific formula?

Within the field of quantum physics, science has come upon an interesting phenomenon: the outcome of an event can be influenced by its viewers. It has taken scientists until now to figure out what shamans have known forever.

The shaman, the "maker of myths" who classically keeps one foot in this world and the other in the spirit world, is not to be confused with the *brujo,* or witch, who dances with evil. Both are powerful. But the shaman holds hands with the Divine, working as a medium between this world's reality and the spiritual realm. He or she charms the Divine into rituals by prayer and song. The shaman's world is of visions and hallucinations, a world of grace and madness.

In Tarapoto, one of the primary cities in Peru for the manufacture and distribution of cocaine, a Frenchman, Dr. Jacques Mabit, began his vision quest by seeking out healers and ayahuasca rituals, looking for a teacher. During his search, a voice spoke to him announcing his future. After six years of research in the Peruvian Upper Amazon, the world's largest coca leaf producing zone, which is also one of the prime consumers of cocaine base, Jacques set up a clinic in Tarapoto in 1992 for research on traditional medicines and for curing cocaine addicts and other drug abusers through ayahuasca shamanism. He called his center Takiwasi.

These days there is an incredible need to keep your immune system strong. Allopathic medicine has confirmed that ayahuasca and other Sacred Power Plants can do just that. According to some healers in Mexico, Ecuador, and Peru, these Sacred Power Plants might even effect a cure for AIDS.

Within the mythologies handed down to us from the mountains of the Andes to the jungles of the Amazon is the same prognostication: we have come full circle. We are now witnessing a move back to the magic and etherealness of our ancestors and the rebirth of shamanism. It is in this realm that we shall ultimately heal all our wounds, for it is here that the soul, the body, and the mind are one and can be cured as a whole, rather than in parts.

In the last five hundred years our focus on industrialization, technology, and "progress" has moved us away from our source. As for me, I have taken a giant step backward, together with the knowledge of the present, to the almost-forgotten medicine and curative powers of the plants and to the healers who work through nature to cleanse the body and who, by divining the plant spirits and the gods, help us connect with the universal life force carried within each of us and so purify the soul. The more each and every one of us, throughout the world, understands this principle, and the sooner we realize that any sickness of the body, mind, or spirit is within the ether that we all share, the more likely the human race will begin to live in health, peace, and harmony.

THE QUEST

Twenty-one years ago, under a rain-swept shop canopy on Amazonas Street in downtown Quito, a wet gringo shouldered into some shelter. "Tourist?" I asked. We were standing so close it would have been uncomfortable to stand there much longer in silence. He studied me for a few seconds before deciding to speak.

"No, I've been comin' here to Quito a couple months a year for the last twelve years." He explained that he was by profession a Louisiana schoolteacher, but three months out of the year he came to Ecuador to search for gold in the Andes.

"How's it going?" I asked.

"It's been gettin' better every year. Last year I was really close—almost found it," he said exuberantly.

What a strange statement, I thought. "Almost? How do you know when you've almost found it?" I asked him.

"I've got a map!" he proudly stated.

I wish I had a map, I thought.

"What brings you here?" he asked me.

Why I would go into the details of my quest I do not know, but I found myself explaining to this gold-hunting Louisiana schoolteacher that I had come looking for a shaman. I felt silly using the vernacular *shaman,* but *curandero,* the correct term for a healer in South America, is way too confusing for the ordinary tourist. Besides, gringos have been telling the curanderos that they are shamans for so long now that many refer to themselves that way.

4

"I came down by land three months ago, through Mexico and Central America to Colombia, and finally to Quito. I've been traveling with Roberto here, from Venice, California." I turned to my friend. "Roberto, this is—what did you say your name was?"

"I didn't, but it's Joe," the schoolteacher said, extending his hand.

I had met Roberto back in Tucson a couple of months earlier, when his name was still Robert. I was to be the photographer for an expedition to the Amazon that Robert had organized. Of the six people who were supposed to be in his party, I was the only one who showed up. My first meeting with Robert came with a knock on my hotel room door; I opened it to a man with long, platinum-blond hair, a chest puffed out like a strutting rooster, and eyes the size of chicken eggs: "You must be Robert."

He reached up high with his right hand, pulling an imaginary train whistle, and yelled, "Whewwwwwww!" After quick introductions, he changed my name: "Dude," he said, holding his palm up looking to slap mine in a high-five salute. Roberto and I decided to continue with the expedition despite the absence of the rest of our party. During the next two months that we traveled together I heard my name, Alan, only enough times to jog my memory. And when we walked across the border into Mexico, he changed his name, too. From that point on he was Roberto. "When in Spain," he shrugged.

Joe the schoolteacher reached into his back pocket, pulling a business card from his billfold. "I don't know who this is," he drawled. "I got it several months ago and still have it. Don't know why I even kept it. Maybe I'm supposed to give it to you. Anyway, here it is."

I liked the way he considered there must be some reason why he saved the card, especially since this was 1992, a year before publication of *The Celestine Prophecy,* the New Age cult classic that popularized the term *synchronicity.* The card was printed in color with a busy logo in the upper left-hand corner that depicted a bird in a heart outline and an eye with a lit candle in the pupil. It was the calling card of Dr. Valentin Hampjes, "Scientific Investigator of Medicinal Plants, Psychiatrist, and Neuro-Medicine."

"Must be a subtle way of saying he's a shaman," I said. We chuckled about the card, which I stuck in my shirt pocket. As the rain tapered away, Joe and I bid adieu.

I had not considered that the healer I would be led to would have a business card. Maybe this was a "map" meant for me. Enough odd synchronicities had occurred to me on this journey already that I couldn't shrug this off.

SYNCHRONICITIES

During my travels with Roberto, I began to discern a pattern of synchronicity, a concept that describes meaningful coincidences, first described by Jung, running throughout my life. These synchronicities could manifest in mundane as well as significant ways.

Two months earlier, as Roberto and I waited in a large and overcrowded Guatemala City bus station, a handsome couple entered the moment my turn came to purchase a ticket that would take me onward in my journey. An unusual energy zinged through me when I noticed them there, thirty meters away. "Roberto, I don't know why, but, for some reason I am supposed to connect with those two people." I walked across the room to the bench where they were seated.

The woman's beauty and regal posture took my breath away. Only then did I realize that perhaps they would not understand English. Taking a chance, I said, "Excuse me, but for some reason I am to speak with you. Maybe you know why?" The man translated my English to his partner, and we continued conversing as she surveyed me. They were brother and sister, from Mexico, on their way home, he told me.

The woman finally spoke. "What do you do?"

"I'm headed to the Amazon to study shamanism."

She smiled, then explained, "I study sorcery in San Louis Potosi, in Mexico. When you have finished your studies in the Amazon, I invite you to come stay with us to learn sorcery. We have a large ranch." She wrote the address down for me. "Of course, you know you cannot have sex for five years when you take this path. It has been three years for me now. Can you do this?"

I was impressed, embarrassed, bewitched, and probably blushing from that statement. She had read my mind.

"It has been two years for me," I lied. It had been only eighteen months, but rounding up to two years nudged me nearer to her bed.

In Calle, Colombia, I watched a man release a guinea pig at a betting pool. It ran down a lane and into a tiny door cut into an upside-down plastic dog-food bowl. There were about fifty of these bowls forming a horseshoe pattern at the end of a twenty-meter-long guinea pig drag strip. The object of the game was to place your money on the bowl you believe the guinea pig would enter. An odd sensation came over me as I played this game. I felt what I call a "knowing," in which I was shown exactly which bowl the animal would choose. Holding my hand out in front of me, I allowed it to be guided to the correct bowl and then placed the change on top. The pig was released and, quite matter-of-factly, sauntered into my chosen bowl.

Roberto saw me yelling, "Yes! Yes!" and collecting the money. "What's happening, Dude?"

I explained how I had received this information.

"It's just coincidence, Dude."

"No, Roberto. It happened just as I told you."

He still refused to accept it, so I told him I would do it again. I held my hand out like a divining rod. Nothing came. I waited. Nothing. It was sort of embarrassing, and so I became a bit agitated. There I was, angry and frustrated, my hand full of change stretched out in front of me, waiting for some otherworldly guidance so I could place a bet. This was ridiculous. Worse, however, was seeing Roberto smirking in the background. The very idea of getting a message this way had to be absurd. But there I was with my arm stretched out, looking like something from *The Return of the Mummy*, hoping something would happen.

I realized that not only was this the first time I had ever called this energy to me but that I had even asked something of it. I quieted my mind and centered myself. Sure enough, after only two or three minutes, it came. Or at least I thought it did. I followed the sensation and moved toward the left side of the lineup of fifty bowls, allowing my hand to place the change on top of the specific one I was guided to. The guinea pig was released. It scurried down the lane to the opposite side of where I had placed my money, stuck its head in the door, then stopped, turned around and marched straight across to the other side, directly into my bowl.

"Yes! Yes!" I yelled, and turned to see Roberto covering his gaping mouth with his hand. Still, I was shocked and stunned. What this experience signified to me was that the energies, spirits, angels, or whatever it was coming to me could be called in. I had never considered that possibility. And it also meant that these same energies were also communicating with the animals.

Glancing back over my life I now see that even during my childhood similar odd events occurred, and at the time I had no realization they contained any significance. Now, with sixty years of experience and being a grandfather, I see things a little more clearly. The years have brought more to me than just perspective; the Light is better.

Remembering my childhood in the foothills of the Appalachian Mountains, I see a child onto which much magic was bestowed. At nine years of age, I was sauntering down Central Street when I was rained on by baby frogs. I looked around and quickly noticed that it was only within my fifty-foot radius that this was happening. I was alone.

A few years later, when my sister was sick, I crept downstairs late at night because something told me to go to her. As I neared her bed, she opened her eyes.

"Alan, what are you doing?" she quietly asked me.

"I don't know, Carla, but I just feel that if I could put my hands near you, move them over your body for a few minutes, I could make you feel better. Is that okay?"

"Yeah, okay."

"Where does it hurt?" I remember asking her.

As she placed her hands on her stomach to indicate where her pain was located, I began moving my hands lightly over the area and thinking about taking away her hurt. I remember having the feeling that I was watching myself do this from a distance—seeing a little boy healing her and watching the healing energy radiate in his hands. After only five minutes I asked her, "Do you feel better?" And in that rich southeastern Kentucky twang of hers she replied, "Why, yes, I do. Thank you, Alan. I do feel better now. I do. You made it go away." In the innocence of youth, she wasn't amazed, and neither was I.

One day, coming home from playing on the mountain, as I stopped to allow my brother to catch up, a strange feeling came over me that I must look under my left foot. Beneath my foot was a rock buried in the ground. I had to dig it up, as only the surface of the rock was exposed. I dug it out with my foot, kicked it over, and it was hollow but full of minerals and crystals—a geode. I was awed by the magical way it was delivered to me.

DR. VALENTIN HAMPJES

The complicated imagery on the calling card of Dr. Valentin Hampjes that the Louisiana schoolteacher had given me remained fixed in my mind, so I decided to phone him. He invited Roberto and me to his home in Tumbaco, a small community twenty miles outside of Quito. We arrived at the home of the good doctor, a cottage nestled at the end of a dirt and cobblestone alley, on a Friday morning. Surrounding the whitewashed brick home were dozens of columnar San Pedro cactus plants, some over six feet tall with several branches. In the center of his front yard was a heart carved out of grass two meters in diameter, rimmed by flowers, and in the center was a huge cactus. We knocked on the door and were greeted by a bearded man of about fifty-five with silver hair and laughing, mischievous eyes. He invited us in.

Valentin spoke fluent Spanish as well as his native German, and intoned his English somewhat like an East European count. His eyes and mouth were constantly smiling in that Freudian "I perceive everything" way, especially when he was puffing on his tobacco pipe, that mannerism perhaps coming from his having received a doctorate in psychiatry and neurology in Vienna, Austria. On the south wall of his home was an altar covered in fresh and dried flowers, with every deity imaginable represented by statuettes, photos, and postcards. He even had a living enlightened master, Sai Baba, contained there in a frame on the altar. To the right of the altar, above the door to his private medical and massage room, was a poster of the Virgin Mary in blissful

11

repose. From the look of all these icons it was clear that Valentin was not the type of shaman to leave anything to chance.

We spent the morning discussing his perceptions of healing through curanderismo. Valentin primarily works with San Pedro, the columnar, psychotropic, mescaline-containing cactus that grows in the Andes. He believes it to be a superior medicine to ayahuasca, a boiled cocktail of a vine and leaf growing in the jungles of the Amazon and also very psychotropic. However, Valentin lives in the Andes, where ayahuasca is not easily available. In my twenty years of apprenticing to the Sacred Power Plants it has been interesting to note that every healer I have ever met has professed that the plant they have the most access to is always the one holding the most power.

Dr. Valentin Hampjes was a very wise and spiritual man, although a bit overly religious in a somewhat exaggerated way. He recognized the healing potentials inherent in allopathic medicine as well as shamanism and would choose one form of medicine over the other to produce the desired results depending on the situation. Lying on the coffee table in front of him was a hardbound copy of a book he had written, *Shamanismo—Extasis of Shamanic Consciousness*. This had been written to justify his having being given a license by the Ecuadorian government to administer entheogens, the sacred plants that engender a psychotropic effect and assist you in realizing the "Divine within," and more importantly, to pass along the knowledge of the use of these plants. A quick glance through the book showed that his roots were also firmly entrenched in Krishna consciousness, of which he was a devotee.

He spoke to me of activating the healer within through the use of the Sacred Power Plants. The wisdom held within these plants can locate the specific malady of a person, whether it be spiritual, emotional, physical, or some combination thereof. If the illness is physical, the body's response or immune system gets activated. If the illness is psychological or spiritual in origin, the patient can be shown, through visions and hallucinations while under the influence of San Pedro or any of the other Sacred Power Plants, when and where the errors were made. In many cases the manifestation of an illness is based in unhealed traumas to the soul; these can lead to psychological imbalances that can ultimately manifest as physical symptoms. If we allow the spirit of the plants to show us why the disturbances exist or where they come from, we can begin to heal ourselves. "You can feel the psychotropic medicines moving through your body, lingering in areas that need attention, activating the immune system to rectify the problem," he explained. "Occidental medicine treats the symptoms, and so our immune system is not activated, it remains asleep."

In speaking with Valentin I learned that it is essential to get the ego out of the way so that healing can take place. One method of accomplishing this is by ingesting the Sacred Power Plants. Sometimes we are granted a vision, which Valentin considers a gift of grace and not to be confused with the many hallucinations coming to you during your journey. However, the mind can manufacture projections of events you have refused to take lessons from or have given little significance to. "This is a hallucination of great value," Valentin explained. "It may come in metaphorical form, so it is essential to pay attention. Visions render knowledge directly from the spirit world and are quite rare."

At the end of our visit, Valentin invited us to return the next day at noon for his weekly San Pedro ritual. His pre-ceremonial advice was to fast upon awakening Saturday morning. Additionally, he gave us a long list of herbs we were to purchase in the Quito market, including several herbs that he would steep in a fifty-gallon container all night long. He asked us to bring fresh-cut flowers for the altar, as well.

Roberto and I arrived on Saturday afternoon, having fasted according to Valentin's instructions. As a result of my conversations with various people in Quito about the upcoming San Pedro ceremony, seven other curious, adventure-seeking tourists from various parts of the globe decided to join us. Upon our arrival we found candles burning on the altar and the smell of incense filled the room. It was early in the afternoon, and Valentin used this time for personality checks, determining the variety of profiles he would have to take into consideration during the evening's ingestion of San Pedro. Each person was asked about their drug history, religious beliefs, what medications they may be on and for how long, what they hoped to gain from participating in the ritual, were there any major physical conditions to be taken into account, and had anyone a history of mental illness and how it had been classified. In general, he was searching for any clues as to possible abnormal behaviors, whether emotional, physical, or spiritual, that might surface while under the influence of the San Pedro medicine. He was especially interested in anyone who had long-term psychiatric problems. Someone who is not balanced in waking reality could certainly have problems with an entheogen. When he questioned me, my responses centered on the energies and synchronicities I had been receiving. I told him that as far as I could tell it seemed as if Spirit were guiding me. He listened, smiling "hmmm" while puffing at his pipe.

We found comfortable seating on benches with cushions that had been placed against the walls of the room, and Valentin instructed us on the proper behavior to maintain during the ceremony.

"When you begin to feel the medicine you must not try and keep your rational mind in focus. This only makes it more difficult. Relax and allow the medicine to move through your body. Ego has no place here. The more you try to hold, the more the medicine will fight you. Get out of its way as quickly as possible. You may see images presented as if on a television screen. Try not to think on them tonight. You will have ample time for that in your reflections tomorrow. If you see something from your past or present, even your future, and it makes you happy or sad, you may laugh or cry if you wish but do not allow yourself to become too entrenched in it. Do not wallow in it. Allow it to pass. Validate it, but do not try and maintain it. Also, if you become frightened and it is necessary that I take your hand and help you through this, I will do so. But remember, 'Yea, though I walk through the valley of the shadow of death, I will fear no evil, for thou art with me.' If you can manage to get through this darkness alone until you find yourself on the other side, back in the Light, you will have become a stronger person for it. However, if there come images you feel you absolutely cannot deal with, simply call me or either of my two apprentices, Mohita or Muridunga, and we will come to sweep them away.

"Please do not converse here in this room," he continued, "as it disturbs not only the others, who may be deeply involved with their personal work, but you must also realize that it prevents you from getting the information you need. Conversation is of the mundane reality and works on a different part of the brain, defeating one of the purposes of the medicine by distracting you from the messages you might otherwise receive. So if you feel you must talk, if you simply cannot keep silent, please go outside."

Someone asked, "Should we be thinking of anything, or have some kind of focus as the San Pedro is taking effect?"

"Bueno," responded Valentin. "At times it is good to focus your thoughts on something you want to have insight into, for to empty your mind of all thoughts is a difficult task to master. And so, no matter how you prefer to approach the ecstatic state, remember: There is a song from North America that goes something like this: 'You can't always get what you want, but if you try, sometimes you may find, you get what you need.'" And with this he laughed that big, semi-hysterical, head-tilted-back laughter that I later grew accustomed to and loved.

We were curiously silent as Valentin turned out the lights and lit candles on the altar, filling the room with the smoke from mapacho tobacco. His two apprentices, Mohita and Muridunga, also Krishna devotees, burned holy wood, *palo santo,* and allowed its smoke to fill every crack and crevice of the house. They were purifying the ceremonial space just as is done with sage in the Native American ceremonies in North America. Valentin had changed into white clothing and, kneeling on the floor in front of the altar, began to pray. He blew smoke from his pipe onto the floor, crossing himself before each exhalation, and then blew smoke to the north, south, east, and west. His prayers continued for five hours, ultimately testing our perseverance.

"When is he going to give us the San Pedro?" whispered one of the guests.

"How much longer?" uttered another voice.

"Soon," I said, guessing it couldn't be much longer.

Then the apprentices rose, and together with Valentin blew tobacco smoke into the bottle of San Pedro, the glass it would be poured into, and another bottle of very dark, almost black liquid.

"The tobacco smoke assures that no negative energies have hidden away," he explained. "If so, the smoke purifies them."

Next he poured tobacco juice into a small glass and walked over to me. "And so, we too must also be purified."

I heard another person whisper, "Does he mean we are going to first drink tobacco juice?"

"Drink this, Alan," said Valentin, offering me the glass.

"Tobacco juice? But won't this make me throw up?" I was confused.

"We hope so," and he laughed. "It will clean out your stomach and act as a catalyst for the San Pedro. Please go outside, either to the rear or the front of the house. And try and avoid throwing up on my cactus plants."

Taking the glass, I jokingly motioned him to open the front door and get out of my way. Obviously, as soon as I drank this it was going to come right back up, and with much more force. We laughed as he opened the door. I swallowed some, and the expected result came. Each person drank their dark brown venom and found their way outside as their stomachs dictated, returning pale and clammy to an awaiting cup of room-temperature *Ilex guayusa* tea. Half an hour later, our stomachs settled, we were given an equal amount, approximately 150 milliliters, of San Pedro. The flavor was just as wicked. We waited. Valentin had cooked it the entire day with no additives—just pure, unadulterated San Pedro cactus. A dose for one person was the distance between your elbow to the knuckles of your closed fist of this spiny, columnar cactus, which was cooked, condensed, and prepared so that you could swallow it in one big gulp.

The San Pedro cactus, *Trichocereus pachanoi,* is one of the Sacred Power Plants and therefore not only is an aid to vision but a powerful medicine as well. It is not simply a source of mescaline, the psychotropic alkaloid that resides in the cactus from the skin inward, about one-eighth of an inch. Many have come to understand where that alkaloid is and cut away the inner portions of the cactus, leaving only a very small percentage of the plant for consuming. This method removes the synergy from the plant, taking its life force out of balance and negating its inherent medicinal attributes (see appendix 1 for a more detailed explanation). It replaces the visionary with pure hallucination. This sophomoric endeavor strips the plant of a portion of its essence, or soul, and transposes the plant's energy into something it was never meant to be, much like the way cocaine is manipulated from the leaves of the coca bush.

The flavor of San Pedro, not much better than the tobacco juice, did not immediately induce vomiting. We resumed our seats on the benches placed around the room and waited for the effects to take hold.

SAN PEDRO

As the San Pedro slowly worked its way through our bodies, Valentin recounted some of his personal history to us.

"I came to the jungles of Pucallpa, Peru, almost twenty years ago from Vienna, where I had been a successful resident surgeon in an Austrian hospital. I had become very frustrated with allopathic medicine, especially its method of treating symptoms rather than the whole person. I was not a spiritual man. In fact, I believed in the logic inherent in science. The afterlife was a concept for the uneducated, I thought. During this time, a very dear friend of mine was diagnosed with incurable cancer and given only a few months to live. As his friends and I believed completely in the validity of modern medicine, we accepted this verdict and decided to give him a going-away party. Following the party, we never saw him again and assumed he had literally gone away to die.

"Approximately three years later I was on call at the hospital. I looked down to the end of a long corridor and thought I saw what must have been the ghost of this man. I stared at this apparition for what seemed like many minutes, frozen in thought. The apparition began moving toward me. I was shocked. I had never seen a ghost or spirit before. In fact, I did not believe in such trivia. I realized I must be hallucinating, and that, too, was frightening for me. It came closer and closer, until I saw it very clearly. It was the ghost of my friend who had died of cancer three years earlier. It walked directly up to me and spoke: 'Hello, Valentin.' I thought I might collapse. Even then I did not comprehend what was happening. I reached out to touch it, thinking my hand must surely go right through it, but it did not. He was alive! My dear, dead friend was alive!

"I was extremely happy to see him, as you can imagine. I asked him what had happened as we thought him dead all these years. He spoke of a journey into the jungles of Peru to see the healers there. They had cured him with their plants and shamanism. He told me of the spirit world and of magical healing songs, called *icaros*. He explained how he had taken a psychotropic medicinal vine called ayahuasca. He related concepts that, were they not coming from a man I deeply respected and knew should be dead of cancer, I would never have believed.

"He shook my whole belief system, my complete foundation. I spent many months afterward rethinking my philosophy of life. This, of course, also affected my approach to medicine. It changed everything. I no longer felt comfortable performing a surgery or prescribing a medicine simply because I could. I began searching for the roots of illness. This method brought me consolation but was not met with the same outlook by the hospital administration. I ultimately concluded that I could no longer pursue healing in just an allopathic way. I was frustrated with my work anyway, so I resigned from the hospital and traveled to Mexico, foolishly searching for Carlos Castaneda and his maestro, Don Juan."

Valentin laughed heartily at himself as he said this, then asked if anyone was yet beginning to feel the effects of the San Pedro. When no one answered, he continued his story.

"I then traveled to Peru, where I began my studies in shamanism, or more correctly, *curanderismo*. Please do not forget, this was over twenty years ago, and traveling to Peru was not a simple affair at that time. I apprenticed with many different jungle curanderos, among whom was a very powerful and spiritual man, Don Jose Fatima, of Pucallpa, Peru, a true healer and ayahuasquero."

At this point Valentin sensed the medicine's effects beginning to work on us and moved to the altar.

"As a newborn child first enters the world of light, breathing its first air, we must never take that light away by extinguishing it with our breath." And then, with a quick flick of his wrist, he snuffed out the candles and said, "It is interesting to note that it is in this darkness, under the influence of the San Pedro, that we begin to *see*. The light reflecting off the surfaces of this reality tends to keep us here."

Almost an hour had passed since we had drunk the medicine. I felt a heat spreading throughout my system and my palms started to sweat. Muridunga began singing and was immediately joined by Valentin. As we became accustomed to the phrasing of the song, everyone participated. Finger and hand drums were passed around the room. The effect of the voices, along with the ever-increasing cadence and intensity of the percussion, allowed every song to flower into a cathartic, emotional expression. We continued singing for a few hours.

It was three o'clock in the morning now and so dark in the room that I couldn't see my hand in front of my face. I thought my energy must be fueled by the passion of the music and its participants, but certainly it must also be coming from the medicine, but I could not be sure. Having had experiences with psychotropic mushrooms and LSD, I always measured their strength visually, from the character of the scenery. But here, I was feeling the medicine in my system without the benefit of any light source, so there was no such measuring stick.

I decided to move outside. Standing there in Valentin's front yard, I needed to step closely by another man in order to pass him. As I did this, I not only felt, but glimpsed my aura passing through his and re-enter me as I stepped around to his other side, sharing for a second or two the same space with his aura. At that moment I felt like I had been washed by a rainbow. He looked back at me with one of those "My God!" type of expressions, and before I could finish saying, "Did you feel that?" he was already responding, "Whoa!" I knew then the medicine had its hand on me.

Valentin joined us outside and asked to speak with me. "Alan, I would like it if you could help me please."

Without knowing what he wanted me for, I quickly stated that I would be glad to do anything I could for him.

"Thank you, Alan. I want to build a center for the children of the streets, the orphans, in the mountains of Vilcabamba."

"Of course you do, but I don't know how I can help you, Valentin. I don't even understand exactly why I am here." I hadn't expected anything so grand as what he was asking of me. I thought he was simply going to ask me to help plant an herb garden or something.

"Excuse me for asking, but why do you want to build this orphanage?" I could tell from his expression I must have looked like a hooked fish and, certainly, he had another good story for me.

And so he began: "A few years ago, a group of medical doctors and I heard that the Holy Mother, the Virgin María, had appeared to the villagers in the mountains near Caracas. We decided to journey there together in the hopes that we, too, might also witness this. When we arrived, the entire valley was covered in tents. Many people had come. We were able to speak with a few of those who had witnessed the Holy Mother, and we realized another sighting would be very unusual. Nevertheless, we too pitched our tents in anticipation of a possible reappearance. We remained there for a few days while many people gathered up their belongings to leave. One evening, as we were talking, she came. We were all just standing there, we doctors, and we witnessed. As you might imagine, we all cried. It was a very emotional scene. We made a pact with one another that evening there in the field: that for the rest of the time we have here on this Earth we shall dedicate it to saving the children. Although I am a doctor as well as a curandero, these things are now secondary. This is why I want to build the orphanage in Vilcabamba."

"That's a beautiful reason. I would be happy to help you, but how?"

"Thank you, Alan. Providence surely brought you to me. Don't think about how you may help now; it will come to you. And Alan, you are correct. You do have a guardian spirit with you. However, it is not one, but three. Tonight I have seen them."

I beamed. "So many miraculous things have happened to me—strange, unexplainable things—both before I left for this trip and during it. It is as if I am being led. I am just trying to keep out of the way so they continue."

"I can see that. You must tell me more of your journey later," he said.

"Valentin, to build an orphanage will take some time. Money has to be raised, and then there's the construction."

"No, we must do this right away. We do not have the time."

"What do you mean, 'We do not have time'? I don't understand."

"Oh, Alan, surely you know, don't you?"

As much as I wanted to tell him that I did, I felt slightly embarrassed, as I had no idea what he was talking about.

"I guess I don't, Valentin. Know what?"

He began a long, impassioned speech about the predictions of Nostradamus and other prognosticators of doom. I listened, intently at first, but as I felt confident from the San Pedro I knew I could not and would not subscribe to the same vision of our future. Eventually I interrupted him and asked, "Valentin, exactly when do you believe this is going to happen?"

"I am sure it will come around the year 2000."

This was distressing to me, not because I was bothered by his forecast, as I didn't believe it anyway, but because he did.

"I don't believe that at all," I told him. "I think the world is becoming more aware all the time. I prefer to believe that we will continue, and that the planet has turned many corners toward that direction. Besides, as you are a very powerful man, Valentin, for you to even think those types of thoughts let alone voice them, which is worse, is to give power to their manifestation. For example, I refuse to mention the name of . . . the devil, and I hesitate to say it here for you now, just to underscore my point, because I believe to do so feeds that energy, it gives it life. And you . . . you are a healer. It is so much more important that you not do so because you have more personal power. Do you understand what I am saying?"

Valentin put his pipe in his mouth and drew in, smiling back at me, and said, "Hmmm . . . Let's return inside to the ritual, shall we? We'll talk more later, Alan."

During the San Pedro ritual, Valentin would occasionally call one or another of his clients in the ceremony to sit on a tree stump placed in front of his altar for a healing. He took a set of palm leaves called a *shacapa* (or *suriponga*) from the side of the altar and began by blowing mapacho tobacco smoke at them for purification of any possible negative energy. This was followed by a misting of *agua florida,* in which Valentin first sipped the liquid and then pressure-sprayed it from his mouth onto the leaves, himself, and the client. Valentin began singing an icaro as he swept the client with the shacapa from his head to his waist. His apprentice Mohita rang tiny bells near and far from the person's ears to realign any misaligned audio-neural pathways. When Valentin was finished, he flicked the palm broom shacapa toward the altar to safely discard any energy it had attracted during the cleansing.

After having witnessed this very important aspect of curing during many subsequent ceremonies, we began to call this portion of the ritual *soul dusting.* Over the last twenty-one years, as I became more adept at it, I began noticing an interesting phenomenon: When I place the shacapa on the crown of my client's head to begin the cleansing, I sometimes see dark splotches, or what the curanderos call *manchas,* attached to the soul-body. They seem to be hanging on to the aura.

My focus is on sweeping them away. There are also astral or spiritual parasites that manifest themselves as insects, which mestizo curanderos refer to as *biches,* but in my twenty-one years of apprenticing I have yet to see one of these. I have no doubt they exist, though, as too many other superstitious, mystical, and otherworldly things have stunningly proved themselves to be true.

Apprenticing has been a constant deciphering and weeding through of myth and acknowledgment of the miraculous. I have a difficult time accepting things just because I am told they are true. Normally, I believe that if a divine mystery is not gifted firsthand by the spirit world, I remain skeptical. For this, my growth as a curandero has been slow, but steady and sure. However, I am often reminded of an Emily Dickinson poem:

> *I never saw a moor,*
> *I never saw the sea,*
> *Yet know I how a heather looks,*
> *And what a wave must be.*
>
> *I never spoke with God,*
> *Nor visited in Heaven,*
> *Yet certain am I on the spot*
> *As if the chart were given.*

That first ceremonial night with San Pedro was astonishing. With all the praying and singing, along with the magical effects of the medicine, I felt more spiritually connected than I ever have in my life.

The morning after the ritual, just as the sun was coming up, while still under the hypnotic influence of the San Pedro, a group of us went outside for a glimpse of reality in the light. The darkness of the previous night had given way to an efflorescent bliss within us. We sighed at the beauty of the morning's glimmering colors. Everything was sprinkled with a luminescent mist of dew. Just at that moment, a white horse stuck his head out from around the far corner of Valentin's house.

"Look! A white horse!" someone said in awe. The timing of this, along with the horse being so white and the colors so much more brilliant as a result of the San Pedro, created such a rush of spiritual magic that we were overjoyed.

"Look! It's coming up into the yard!" The horse moved slowly up into the yard and continued across. It was approaching the heart carved into the grass in Valentin's yard.

"It's going into the heart!" This was almost too much beauty to handle. The white horse walked into the very center of the heart and just stood there, looking back at us. We were speechless, certain San Pedro was presenting us with some mystical message, some incredible encapsulation of the night's events. The horse slowly turned around. Its tail was facing us now. We were trying to determine what the significance of this was when, then and there, as we were in complete wonder of the majesty of it all, searching for the "message," the animal took a big dump. Daylight and reality combined, smacking us in the face. I cannot remember when I have laughed so hard and felt so healed.

We returned inside, and Valentin informed us it was now time to continue our cleansing in his backyard. He led us outside, where Mohita was waiting with more tobacco juice. The apprentice drew 6 cc's of the vulgar, murky brown fluid into a needleless syringe and inserted it into our nostrils, injecting first one side, then the other, while we held our breaths. Valentin explained the process as he did this:

"The tobacco juice will drop down into the sinus cavities with only a slight sting and an instant's sensation of drowning. It washes the phlegm out of the cavities, down the throat, and into the stomach. You must then douse your nostrils with fresh water and quickly drink a sixteen-ounce cup of warm guayusa tea. The tea mixes with the tobacco and phlegm in the stomach, producing a purgative reaction. Many of the diseases we have are caused by an excess of phlegm. The phlegm moves throughout your body and eventually settles, attracting toxins. These toxins cause illness. For this reason, curanderismo is concerned with ridding yourself of as much phlegm as possible. It is best to repeat this tobacco remedy three or four times. When you have finished, you will hear your voice as if for the first time, crystal-clear, like a bell."

Tobacco juice treatments are not for everyone, as they can be quite toxic to some people. The First World has been partially brainwashed by all the propaganda around tobacco. We need to understand that this plant, in its unadulterated form, free from chemical additives and grown without pesticides, has been used in a sacred and medicinal manner by every indigenous culture in the world that has ever been introduced to it. It is not tobacco that causes addictions and cancer; it is the 400 or so additives that companies put into it, some of which have even been banned for any other use whatsoever.

A light lashing with stinging nettles followed the phlegm purge. We stripped off our clothes and hosed ourselves down with cold water. Mohita sprayed our bodies with an antiseptic called *seguro,* a mixture of basil, camphor, ruda (rue), and wormwood plants in a base of aguardiente, the moonshine made from the distillation of sugarcane; then he whipped our entire bodies with the sprigs of *ortega,* stinging nettles. While many impurities are excreted through our pores, we still build up toxins between the upper two layers of our skin, which is why Valentin encouraged us to endure the ortega beating. The skin is punctured thousands of times by the tiny barbs, allowing the toxins to escape. Again, this cleansing does not come easily. Your body feels like it's on fire, and small red welts begin to rise, which stay with you for the next hour, then slowly fade away. This is followed by a warm herbal bath that has been steeping the entire night.

"This is the final cleansing," said Valentin. "You have been thoroughly cleaned, inside and out, and so it is important not to put any synthetic soaps, shampoo, or toothpaste into your system for the next twenty-four hours."

Thus began my teachings on San Pedro under Dr. Valentin Hampjes. Thereafter, every Saturday, I bused to his home in Tumbaco. I continued these ceremonies once a week for the next four months.

BREAKING THROUGH BARRIERS

After the first three rituals, I determined that the San Pedro was too weak for me; one dose would bring in no more than energy and colors. For this reason I would always ask to be given a second dose. This was frustrating for Valentin.

"But why do you want such a large dose, Alan?"

"I am not here for homeopathic doses, Valentin. I am physically healthy."

"What are you trying to do, break through some sort of barrier?"

"Exactly." I responded. "I want to *see*."

Valentin's apprentice Mohita had often told me of having been visited by the spirit of San Pedro, a small, pockmarked man, apparently similar to the spirit of peyote. I wanted to see him and other interdimensional things. I thought that because of my First World programming, it would take a healthy dose of the medicine to get me there. Valentin reluctantly poured me a double dose from then on.

When we experience something that cannot be explained in our normal reality, we usually dismiss it, as our eyes are attuned to another version of reality: the waking state, the programmed day-to-day existence, the reality chosen for us and hammered into us. Somewhere around the age of five or six, something tragic but evidently essential happens: the psychological programming begins to set in. Whether this is the direct result of having integrated a basic language or simply a learning of social codes, or both, I really do not know. No doubt, each of these has its effects. You can see it in a child's eyes and in his or her manner and behavior. This conditioning "takes" so well the child even becomes proud of it. And because of the child's inherent competitive nature, this game is unending, continuing into adulthood and beyond, into old age—unless something happens to create a change of awareness. In this way socialization steadily paints itself over our native intuition, and the attunement of our vision is no more.

Our payment for entrance into society is the forfeiture of our sixth sense, which includes intuition and telepathy. We are taught to draw our conclusions from our five senses, as the sixth one is neither tangible nor logical, and therefore we have no method of discerning its existence. Indeed, there are shamans who say that we have many more senses, senses that we have not yet discovered let alone learned how to use.

We live in an empirical world that has slowly and methodically taken away the credibility of our mind's belief in miracles and the ability to suspend our disbelief. It isn't that magic has gone—it's just that we have forgotten how and where to look and listen for it. We have foolishly allowed information to replace intuition. Half-wittedly, we have also removed ritual from our lives. In our search for concise, logical communication, we have spelled near-death to whatever telepathic, extrasensory abilities we human beings once had. We have forgotten that we must continue to allow ourselves to be mystified, that we must remain receptive to knowledge not generally known.

For instance, about thirty years ago, while doing research in a small, mining-town library where I was working, I had an otherworldly experience that could not be explained. I was quietly busy in the back corner of the library, trying to determine which play would be most appropriate to direct in this Bible Belt community. Other than the librarian at her desk near the front door, I was alone.

In telling this story I must backtrack a bit: My uncle, Albert Thomas Shoemaker, was my father figure, as my mother had divorced when I was three years old. Three months earlier I had received a

National Endowment for the Arts grant that had placed me in this small Bible Belt town as its artist-in-residence; right afterward, my beloved uncle, who had been working with Al Capp and Stan Drake as a cartoonist, drawing L'il Abner and Juliet Jones cartoon strips, died in a car wreck in Boston.

And so there I was, sitting quietly, alone in this country library, when a sensation came over me to stand up and begin walking past several stacks of books. The feeling is difficult to describe, as I was spoken to in a way that negated actual words but gave me a "knowing" or clairaudience. I followed this inner voice, passing several stacks, turning left when told to do so, walking between the shelves until the voice told me, "Stop, reach out, and grab a book." Without looking, I did so, pulling down a book with my left hand. Opening it up to the first page, I read: "Dedicated to Albert Thomas Shoemaker." I had never heard of this book. Checking with his immediate family later, it was revealed that several years earlier my uncle had given the author a room in his home in Spain in which to write it.

I continued drinking San Pedro with the good doctor for several weeks and spent my free time in Quito, Ecuador. During one week I kept seeing a very unusual young man playing pool with two of his friends in a local tavern. I sipped a beer and watched him. There was something about him, I did not know for sure, but something was . . . wrong. He wasn't very adept at the game, and perhaps this discomfort was what I was picking up on. He was maybe twenty years old, and from his carriage and demeanor, obviously quite intelligent. However, from his movements around the table, it was clear that something was out of balance with him. At first I thought it was the pool game, but after watching him for half an hour I knew it was something else. But what?

I left the tavern thinking about the young man, and two days later I saw him again, this time at a sidewalk café. I had an opportunity to sit at his table, and as it turned out, we knew some of the same people. Alexander was his name, but he preferred Sasha. He was from Norway. English was among the many languages he spoke. Here on a grant to perfect his Spanish, he had done that in rapid fashion. During our conversation he let me know that he had survived cerebral malaria, sometimes a deadly disease, because the hospitals in Quito had caught it in its early stages. The problem now was his short-term memory. The hospital doctors and specialists knew of no way to completely recover it. The electrical connections—the synapses—had been short-circuited. He could be in the middle of a conversation and forget who he was talking with, the subject, or even where he was. For this brilliant young man, this was his worst nightmare come true: the brain he had trained to understand fifteen different languages and speak seven fluently was no longer functioning properly. He had the stamina to withstand this cosmic joke but nonetheless was in immense inner turmoil over it.

I consulted with Valentin, who was, after all, a neurosurgeon, regarding the young man. The good doctor agreed that his electrical synapses had been overtaxed, and that drinking San Pedro could reconnect them. Sasha agreed to attend a ceremony, and Valentin's instructions to him for the week prior to the ritual were to take a holiday and refrain from all intellectual activity.

I attended the ceremony with Sasha. Three hours after we drank the medicine, Valentin called him to come sit in front of the altar for a cleansing. Icaros were sung, the shacapa was used to soul dust him, and Mohita continually rang tiny bells at various distances from his ears. When they finished with him, he came over and sat down next to me.

"Alan, thank you for bringing me out here. I have my short-term memory back."

"Just like that?" I asked.

"Yes. Valentin said the medicine could bring it back, and it has."

Sasha was rarely amazed. Valentin did exactly what he said he would do, and Sasha completely expected it and immediately accepted it when it happened, just like that.

One evening at Sasha's home I told him a story from my childhood. I was ten years old and spending the night with my friend Charlie. He was on the top bunk bed and I was on the bottom. We decided to play a card game where he would pick a card from the deck, concentrate on it, and I would divine the correct card. I chose the correct card three times in a row, after which Charlie thought the game quite boring, so we went to sleep. Then again, one year before I left Seattle for this shamanic journey, I mentioned this story to my friend Elizabeth and she suggested we try it. This time she was sitting directly in front of me with a deck of playing cards. She chose a card and thought of nothing else. Again I chose the correct card and suit three times in a row.

"Do you think you could do it again now?" Sasha asked.

"I don't know . . . but I think so."

"Alright, I have a deck of cards upstairs in the office. I'll be right back."

While he hopped upstairs and grabbed the deck, I headed down the hallway to the bathroom. Entering the doorway, two images of cards came into my head.

"Sasha," I yelled, "Sasha, have you chosen a card yet?"

"Yes, I have."

Walking back into the living room I said, "Look, I haven't done this in a while and I don't know, this is weird: as I was walking to the bathroom I began getting an image, but it's not of one card, but two. And you have chosen a card, right?"

"Yes, I have."

"Well, I get two cards coming, I don't know why, but . . . I get the nine of clubs and a red jack."

Sasha wasn't even surprised, he just said, "When I first picked up the deck I saw only the bottom card, the nine of clubs. And here is the jack of diamonds. And he took the card off his forehead from under his glasses. "These are the only two cards I have seen." I was impressed, surprised, and amazed. He was very matter of fact, nothing more.

When I jokingly suggested we become bridge partners, he just said, "Alan, that would be cheating."

Four months of drinking the San Pedro medicine with Valentin had left my physical body cleaner than it had been since I was a twenty-year-old. From all the purging, I also felt emotionally cleansed, as I had learned not only to purge myself of the toxins in my stomach, but to allow my psychological self to purge at the same time. As a result, I was glowing. But the time soon came for me to continue my journey.

Every time I glanced at a map of South America, the city of Iquitos would zing in my brain. I felt called to leave the safety of my San Pedro group and explore the upper reaches of the Amazon in search of a maestro who could teach me the mysteries of its principal medicine, ayahuasca. Valentin attempted to persuade me not to leave. He was sure I would fall into the hands of unethical brujos who would slip other dangerous psychotropics into the ayahuasca in order to control me. But my mind was set. The Amazon was calling.

IN SEARCH OF A MAESTRO

I was strolling down a strange street with some person I didn't know. Directly in front of us, a man jumped out from behind a tombstone-shaped sculpture, screamed something in Spanish about a woman, and fired a pistol. The stranger and I dove for cover in opposite directions. The bullet hit me directly in my right temple, blowing my head off. I remember thinking, *I must now be dead because if I die in a dream I must die also in waking reality.* My body was floating in a black void, spinning and spinning, and finally flopped back down onto my two-dollar-a-night cot at the hostel in Baranquilla, Colombia, jolted awake, drenched in sweat.

For a couple of years I interpreted this dream as meaning that I would one day see my death in this manner. Later I understood that this was an important dream—that this "death" was an essential beginning for my apprenticing in shamanism. Or at least I preferred to look at it that way. However, even now as I write this, I am not 100 percent sure my future has not already been forecast.

Deep down into the Colombian Amazon, on the muddy, rust-colored banks of the Putumayo River, lives an old Siona curandero who has been taking care of his tiny village and its assorted illnesses, performing ayahuasca rituals at least once a week, for the past sixty years. It was here I began my studies and it was here I realized I was being called to the ayahuasquero healer's path. Later, I would apprentice with the ayahuasquero Don Juan Tangoa, outside of Iquitos, Peru.

But the signs guiding, affirming, and maintaining my path left no room for doubt as to their authenticity; I would find my maestro and apprentice myself.

Ayahuasca and the other Sacred Power Plants heighten our awareness, opening the doors to the spiritual plane of existence. They guide us to our center, where within each of us sleeps an internal doctor, the healer within, which, once activated, allows us to heal ourselves. These sacred medicines invoke a specific healing response, clearing out physical maladies and alleviating psychological duress from the past, such as ingrained habits and response patterns that have long outgrown their usefulness, allowing us to move on and continue to grow. It is imbibed ceremoniously with the guidance of a skilled curandero who controls the many spirits conjured through the incantation of icaros, the curandero's magical melodies, taught to him literally by the spirits of the plants.

The old Siona curandero in the village on the banks of the Putumayo River poured my first cup of ayahuasca. We sat surrounded by the jungle in a thatched-roof, dirt-floored, open-walled *tambo*. Present at the ritual were eight tribesmen obviously just a couple of generations out of their traditional attire, in various modes of hand-me-down First World clothing—well-worn t-shirts, U.S. imitation jeans, overly abused tennis shoes, flip-flops—along with three shaman-hunting gringos who had shared the ride down the river with me in a fifteen-meter-long dugout canoe.

The other gringos and I had pooled our money in Quito, Ecuador, and headed for Colombia together in search of the entrance to the Upper Amazon via the Rio Putumayo, a narco-trafficking river with the harshest reputation for kidnappings and untimely disappearances. We traveled by bus up and over high mountain passes, on narrow one-lane dirt roads that looked as if they could cave in at any moment. In three days of breathing dust and exhaust fumes and being stopped by the Colombian police for drug searches, we finally found ourselves in the brawling cowboy town of Puerto Asis, Colombia, and the head-waters of the Putumayo. Here were dirt streets, motorcycles reined up outside saloons, and front-row seats to street shoot-outs viewed from our hostel balcony. An English-speaking, gringo-friendly, out-of-work schoolteacher whose son supposedly represented Colombia in fencing for the Olympic games even came up with a brilliant way to introduce our innocence to Puerto Asis, the cocaine Mafia, and the FARC, the Revolutionary Armed Forces of Colombia, the Marxist-Leninist revolutionary guerrilla organization involved in the continuing armed conflict in this country since 1964. He suggested a recorded welcome to its residents, in English, on the local radio station, so I recorded the greeting, simulating as closely as I could Robin Williams in *Good Morning Vietnam!*

"Good morning, Puerto Asis! This is Alan Shoemaker from the United States wishing each and every one of you a fine and healthy good morning. Buenos dias!" This, I'm told, to this day, twenty-one years later, is still played from time to time.

It took two weeks of daily searching to find our fifteen-meter-long dugout canoe and a forty-horsepower motor. We rigged it with curved rebar roof supports to support a black plastic rain tarp and bought enough food to last one month. Four fifty-five-gallon drums of gasoline and a few mechanic's tools rounded out our purchases. We motored out of Puerto Asis by a small tributary and onto the Rio Putumayo, maneuvering into what seemed a fast eleven-mile-an-hour current. It was a shaman hunt, and we were determined to ride this dugout all the way to La Chorrera, Colombia, a Bora-Huitoto-Ocaina village nestled around impassable waterfalls on the banks of the Igara Paraná River.

After solving various engine problems, we eventually motored onto the banks of a tiny Siona tribal village, where we were greeted by some of the native people. We asked to see their curandero.

"Si, señor. He can't see you today. He's drunk."

Drunk? Their healer was drunk? "That's okay, we'd like to see him anyway."

The other gringos followed the man to a thatched-roof hut built on twelve-foot-high stilts for protection from the rising river and wild animals. After arranging for one of the locals to guard our canoe, I, too, climbed the stairs to his house and, for some strange reason, pushed the door open and paused for a moment before going in. I heard a drunken shout of "Jaguar!" then abashedly eased into the room like a clumsy house cat, knocking over a flowerpot in the process, the faces in the small room anxiously staring at me. An old man, apparently their curandero, was sitting on a small stool near a large, screenless window overlooking the village. The hair growing out of his head was silvery and long and lent a haunting effect to a face of sunbaked, cracked mud. I stared at him as the "serene holy man" image that I had conjured up in my mind faded slowly away like the illusion it was, disappearing into the wrinkled tributaries of his face.

It was still early, so the old man asked me to buy him another half-pint of aguardiente, the potent alcohol made from the distillation of sugarcane. He spoke in Spanish, slightly better than mine and quite understandable. He quickly chugged the aguardiente, then agreed to brew a pot of ayahuasca and perform a ritual for us that very evening.

"But don't we have to diet all day?" I asked.

"No, no. Meet me here later. My wife will cook dinner and we go out to the tambo and drink."

"We can eat just before drinking ayahuasca?" I was confused. This was contradictory to the teachings of Valentin.

"Of course we can. Won't you be hungry? She'll make chicken soup. Don't you like chicken soup?" he asked me.

The lessons learned from the Sacred Power Plants come in a variety of ways. It would take working with many different curanderos to dispel my belief that in order to be a healer you necessarily need to also be a perfect human being and that you need to be absolutely impeccable.

Someone made that up, and God bless him. And it does not really matter whether the person is called a *shaman* or a *curandero,* it is the intent behind the word. We have endowed these magnificent healers with concepts of perfection they could not possibly live up to. We have misidentified them as "holy men," and some of them have hopelessly tried to embrace that notion. So much reverence and mystique accompanies the term *curandero* that the person whom it describes has no place to go except to eventually fall off the pedestal on which we have inappropriately placed him or her. The curandero is therefore in a catch-22: we dreamt the idea, and he must therefore try to be it, right? But the curandero can never live up to the adulation reflected on the faces of the gringo. One misstep and he is next thought of as nothing more than a mere charlatan. My first encounter with that old Siona ayahuasquero would shatter the myth of the stereotype and teach me much about what a true curandero is.

We arrived at the curandero's home at 6:00 p.m. as instructed. I spooned away two bowls of soup, the second one going down with only shadowy thoughts of the possible repercussions from not following what I had been taught was the proper diet before a ritual. It was dark when dinner was over, so we grabbed our flashlights, mosquito nets, and hammocks, then followed the old man along a muddy trail deeper into the jungle until we arrived at his ritual hut, a tambo approximately one kilometer from his home. The ayahuasca had been cooking since early afternoon, and the ashes were still warm.

"Has it been cooking long enough?" I asked.

"More than enough time," he assured me.

I was skeptical, but then this was the jungle, and I really didn't know what to expect. From the information I had gathered about ayahuasca, I thought it had to cook at least eight hours, but what did I know? I decided to go with the flow and take his medicine with an open mind, just as I had eaten two bowls of his wife's chicken soup.

I swallowed my very first cup of still-warm ayahuasca, kneeling in respect to the maestro and toasting the ritual for all its spiritual qualities. The flavor was atrocious. He handed us a four-inch piece of peeled sugarcane, instructing us to suck on it to take the flavor away. When he gave me a piece, I remembered Valentin's instructions: "No sugar in any form after taking a Sacred Power Plant." I thought this was one of the many rules you were simply not to break. However, he was the curandero, this was his jungle, and the flavor was sickening, so, as with the chicken soup dinner, I gladly followed his instructions. Then I waited.

An hour passed and I was feeling no effect. The others were obviously under the ayahuasca's influence, walking as if the ground were in the throes of a small earthquake, serenading me with various cacophonous purging noises, melodious frequencies that seemed to dance around me from outside the tambo. The old ayahuasquero slapped his harmonica on his hand, emptying its excess saliva, and rose from his hammock. He had not sung even one icaro, apparently preferring to work with the vibratory sounds of his harmonica. He ambled over to his pot of medicine, squatted down, opened the lid, picked up the coffee cup he used to dose it out, and nodded for me to come join him. I stood and walked over to him. He sat there behind his pot of still-warm ayahuasca, studying me. After a few moments, he tendered another cup and suggested that I might have some resistance to the effects of the first one, that perhaps I had a block. And again, as with his chicken soup and the sugarcane, I refused to allow my own preconceived notions to guide me. I had to go for this; I had to trust my instincts about this initially inebriated, codgy old Siona ayahuasquero. I shot this repulsive fluid past my taste buds into my throat and had no problem accepting his offer to suck on more sugarcane. I waited.

I watched the stars glistening under a half moon. My awareness heightened from listening to the symphony of jungle music blending with the extraordinarily mellifluous notes of these icaros, blown into the harmonica by this crusty curandero. An hour and a half had passed since my first cup, half an hour since my second. When I started to clear my throat, a geyser erupted in the deepest pools of my stomach with such force that I ran out of the tambo, both hands slapped firmly against my mouth, with unstoppable spews of vomit spraying from between my fingers. After about thirty meters I stopped running, removed my hands, and let fly the rest of this unyielding liquid, completely awed by its strength and pressure, which seemed to be gushing forth a meter or so in front of me, over and over again, until my stomach completely emptied its contents.

Suddenly, as I stood hovering over the ground like the hunchback of Notre Dame, I noticed lights out of the corners of my eyes. The ceremonial participants, obviously concerned, surely must have followed me out into the jungle and were now standing all around me because I noticed what must have been the glimmers of their flashlights. I was embarrassed. I must gather my wits and present them with the proper mask, I thought, as I tried to balance myself. I stood up straight, focused my eyes, and to my surprise, witnessed the most unbelievable thing I have ever seen: all the jungle plants in the semicircle of my vision were inhabited by spirits. They were glowing from the inside out! Within the very small plants just off to my left were the spirits of indigenous children, and directly in front of me, at twelve o'clock, large shrubs contained giant, twenty-foot-tall tribal spirits with below-the-shoulder-length hair held with headbands, resplendent in traditional attire: armbands and long robes in a checkered pattern of lime green, cream, and white. I knew that this medicine was a powerful hallucinatory and thought it particularly interesting that my mind would be so detailed as to fabricate their collars in a Nehru fashion.

What was happening to me? Was I hallucinating? Was this a vision? My mind analyzed the various possibilities while my body responded with cold chills running up and down my spine. Just at that moment, the entire group of spirits, eight in all, put their arms out, palms up in a welcoming fashion, and began singing my name. I could hear the soprano and alto voices of the women and children and the deep resonant voices of the men singing beautifully, in harmony, "Alan, Alan, Alan, Alan, Alan . . ." Tears streamed down my face. I had an overwhelming urge to bow down to them in reverence, but instead nodded my head in an honoring gesture of respect as I stood there, consumed and mystified by this magnificent Amazonian vision. In that space it seemed as though the vision lasted ten minutes. Ten minutes I stood there in absolute wonderment, until I finally spoke, thanking them for what they had shown me, explaining that I must return to the tambo and the ritual, promising them that I would never forget what they had shown me.

Maybe now I was beginning to understand, but I was still unsure. *Is this it? Curanderismo? Shamanism? Are there literally spirits of plants, and if they so choose, can they heal you? If we listen, can they teach us?* I had too many things to think about, but they would all have to wait till morning.

When I had quickly run out of the tambo to purge, I noticed no change in my coordination. After purging I had trouble determining when my feet were going to hit the ground. The upper portion of my body, however, was in complete control. The drunken effect seemed to be only in my legs. Perhaps it was just that my feet were the farthest from my eyes and my eyes were then the actual cause of this? Could it be that the farther away objects were, the more likely you would hallucinate on them? And had I been hallucinating everything? That would help explain what I had just seen. But these spirits had sung to me, hadn't they? They even knew my name.

I returned to the ritual, sat down at my place, and was astonished by completely vivid images of jaguars and boas that seemed to emerge from out of nowhere, in utter darkness, ferociously presenting themselves just inches away from my face. Although I was unsure exactly what this was or why it was happening, I decided to suspend my disbelief and perceive it as a bizarre test of bravery. As the jaguar roared directly into my face, I was able to see, in full color, each and every tooth, its tongue, and even down into its throat. Instead of becoming frightened, I decided to appreciate the beauty of the images, for what choice did I have? This was beyond my control. And what if this really was a test of courage? I had learned many years ago to have an admiration for danger, maintaining fortitude in its wake. For the next three hours I was bombarded with visions of the viciousness of the jungle, until the effect of the ayahuasca finally tapered away and the ceremony came to a close.

As many thoughts whirled around in my mind and the visuals slowly melted away, I climbed into my hammock and fell into a deep sleep, awakening with the first light. My companions and I slowly gathered what gear we had and returned to the curandero's home in the village.

One of my canoe partners, Thea, and I openly discussed the night's imaginings. She told me about the curandero's son who had drunk the ayahuasca with us. He had met her down by the stream where she had gone to purge. After splashing some water on her face, she began her return to the thatched-roof tambo, but he was standing in the middle of the trail, blocking her way. She thought nothing of it and continued walking toward him. He didn't move. She stopped directly in front of him and he reached out, placing his hands on her breasts. Thea looked at him and calmly and firmly said, "No," and he moved aside. She returned to the ritual, deeply under the influence of the medicine, and he followed, sitting between us on a small platform. I had occasionally looked over at him during the night, especially when he was making deep roaring sounds like a bull. He seemed to be in a deep trance, his eyes closed.

Thea explained: "During the night, while I was in deep meditation, I sensed he was trying to come to me in spirit form for sex." She was unsure whether this was real but felt strongly enough to erect an other-dimensional wall, not allowing him entry; and it was real enough to mention to me. However, because it revolved around sex, she wasn't completely convinced of its authenticity. Within the ayahuasca state, she believed that had she wanted to allow him into her visions he could have entered her.

I didn't know what was real or imaginary either but thought that perhaps this was a gift from the spirits to her concerning her sexuality. "The only way you will ever know is to ask him," I suggested, realizing I, too, had received a gift of a vision that still needed to be processed. Thea, however, felt too uncomfortable to approach him and a few days later told me, "Alan, I wish I had done as you suggested, because now I will never know."

I, too, thought I would never know, for during the next year of my apprenticeship in curanderismo I was never absolutely convinced of what I had seen that night. The old Siona curandero had plainly told me his medicine contained only the ayahuasca vine, chaliponga, and a few leaves of datura. I believed him, and now I know that the effects of this medicine last only four hours, and the dry, parched-throat feeling coming from ayahuasca overlaced with datura had not been present. Datura is a bush and also grows in tree form, with long, bell-shaped flowers hanging downward. It's an enticingly beautiful plant and in the wrong hands can be deadly when overdosed. It is typically used by brujos and others posing as shamans, as they either don't have knowledge of how to properly prepare ayahuasca, or, if they do, they're too lazy to cook it properly. Datura is loaded with atropine, scopolamine, and hyocyamine, all very dangerous chemicals. In controlled doses it is sometimes ruthlessly used to spike someone's drink, basically turning the person into a zombie so that he follows all your commands, such as giving you his ATM card and pin number.

The old Siona shaman met with us the morning after the ritual, and we traded harmonicas: my new blues harp for his slightly rusty and well-used Colombian one. It was a gift I treasured. He was the first to explain to me that according to legend, the new curanderos would be gringos. And that a little over five hundred years ago the Spanish had come with their diseases and instruments of war and had decimated them, not interested in learning their organic healing methods. The time had now arrived, the beginning of the next five-hundred-year cycle, and the old ayahuasquero could find no one to teach. Even his son, whom he would most like to pass his knowledge to, wasn't interested, he told me. But we gringos are interested—or at least those gringos who have seen and understand the idiocy inherent in the cause-and-effect of the logic systems that we have created and implemented in this world. The shamanic world is a mystical world, and we gringos have been educated well enough to respect what was left behind and to try to save what parts of it we can before it is lost forever. The missionaries have come with their First World financing, and they float planes and set up churches in the deepest reaches of the jungle, bringing with them their God, their ethics, and their morals. They have convinced the mestizo and indigenous peoples, through gifts of clothing, medicine, and money, that the traditional medicine from their grandfathers is nothing more than superstitious folklore. Now the newly attired children prefer to swallow a pill and worship a God their people previously knew nothing of. They are no longer interested in preserving their heritage.

The old Siona healer dishearteningly continued, telling me of his son and various other apprentices who had given up. Besides the competition from the missionaries, there is the lure of the free clinics floating up and down the Putumayo and established in various pueblos, dispensing antibiotics and parasite medications. It is much easier to pop a pill than to endure the difficult tests and trials that one must face during a shamanic apprenticeship. The plant diets are designed to help a person connect with the spirits of the plants and to develop new healing capabilities, vision, and sight; they require much time in solitude and a strict dietary regime. For this reason they are physically and psychologically strenuous, and many apprentices would not return after they began the various diets required of them in order to master a Sacred Power Plant. Some of the tree doctors require strict diets of ninety days and more, alone in the jungle, before you can drink or work with them, the old shaman explained. He was quite sad that his knowledge wouldn't be passed on through his own tribe and bloodline, and it was in this sense that he fully understood the significance of handing me his harmonica. He was passing something very special on to me in the hope that I might continue the unbroken chain—that I might one day become this new curandero, the "gringo shaman," and therefore a vessel maintaining the ancient knowledge he treasured and hoped would survive the passage into this new age that he, from time to time, saw fleeting glimpses of as it floated by on the Putumayo.

After meeting this beautiful and wise Siona healer, I realized that my methods of healing would evolve. I hoped I would learn to direct my energies toward asking questions of my patients before and following rituals, guiding them through self-inquiries, helping them recognize and work with their own internal healing energies.

When we left the following morning, the parting was bittersweet. I informed the old ayahuasquero I would try to return, but he and I both knew the possibility of this happening was slim. However, both of us realized that this was also one of the many beginnings of the five-hundred-year legend he had shared with me. Moreover, I left knowing I had seen and felt real, earthy curanderismo, unadulterated by First World concepts and unadorned by all its rules, which I had sacrificed so much to learn and was now trying so hard to break.

Amidst the bedlam of the Putumayo exists a key to healing. In a tiny, dirty village on the muddy, rust-colored banks of this dangerous river lives a sometimes drunken and always sad ayahuasquero who showed me that the world's rain forests and the ancient practices of healing that had evolved there are not a sham. There does exist the possibility of discovering a cure for the maladies of the world. It just may be that it doesn't come in a pill or a bottle; it may not even be something that you can touch with your hands. Maybe it's an ethereal magic that will never be glimpsed under a microscope. Perhaps the future of healing is in access to and communication with another plane of existence.

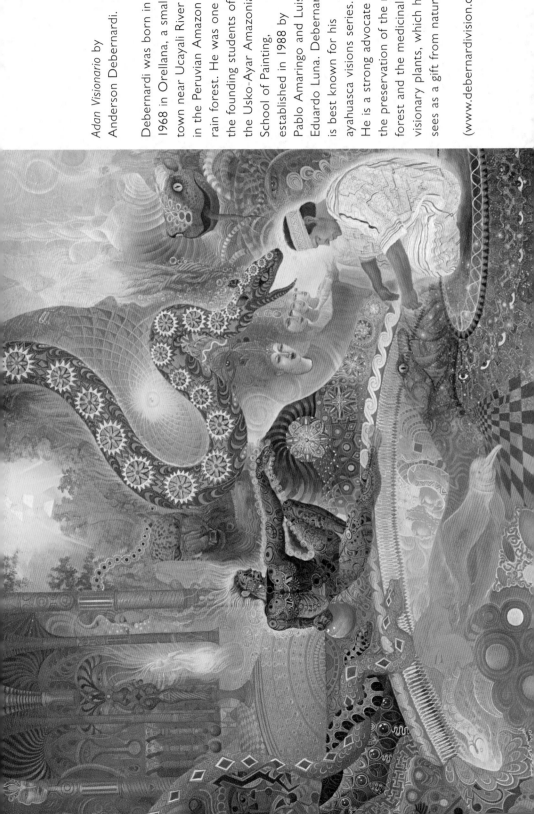

Adan Visionario by Anderson Debernardi.

Debernardi was born in 1968 in Orellana, a small town near Ucayali River in the Peruvian Amazon rain forest. He was one of the founding students of the Usko-Ayar Amazonian School of Painting, established in 1988 by Pablo Amaringo and Luis Eduardo Luna. Debernardi is best known for his ayahuasca visions series. He is a strong advocate for the preservation of the rain forest and the medicinal and visionary plants, which he sees as a gift from nature.

(www.debernardivision.com)

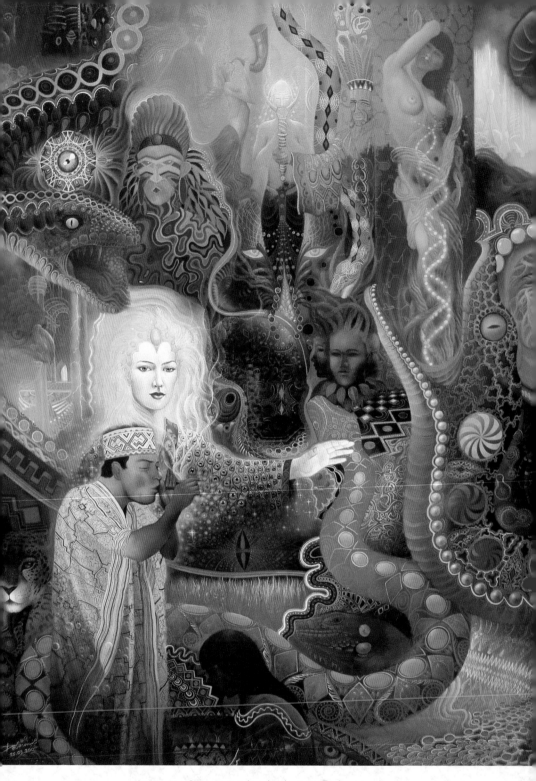

Iniciacion Shamanica by Anderson Debernardi

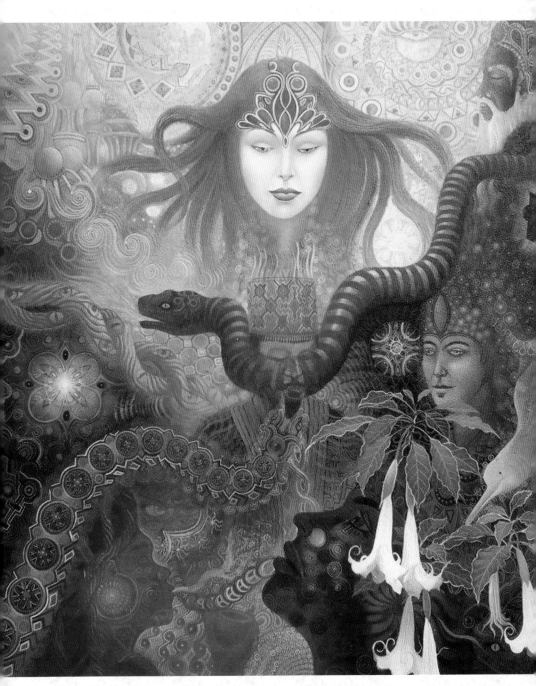

Trance Shamanico by Anderson Debernardi

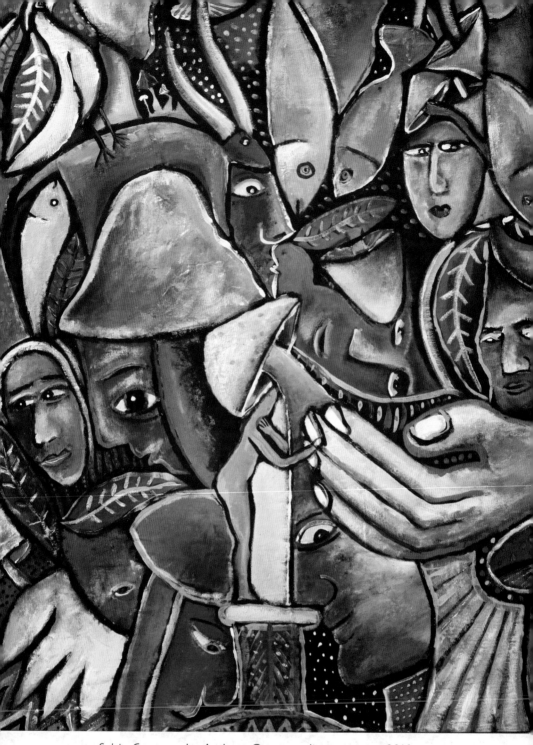

Salvia Ceremony by Andrew Osta, acrylic on canvas, 2010.
Following an eight-month ayahuasca apprenticeship in Peru, Ukrainian-born
Osta created a series of paintings capturing aspects of his experience with the
ceremonial/visionary inner world.
(www.andrewosta.com)

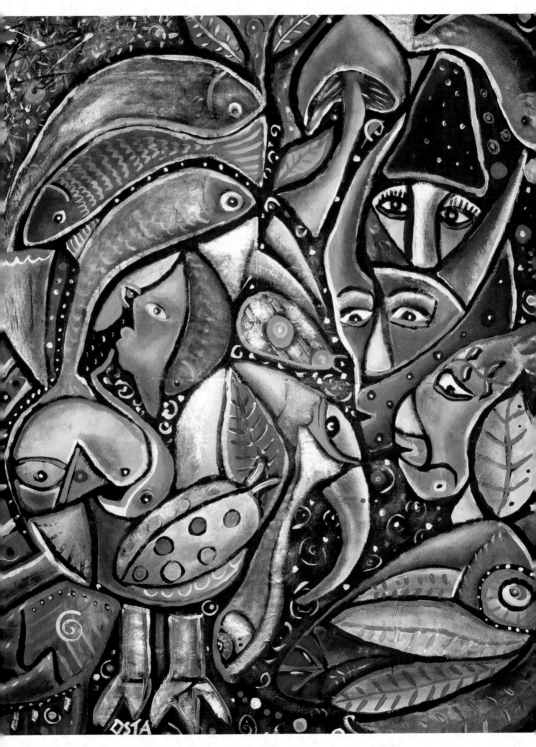

Russian Fairytale by Andrew Osta, acrylic on canvas, 2010.

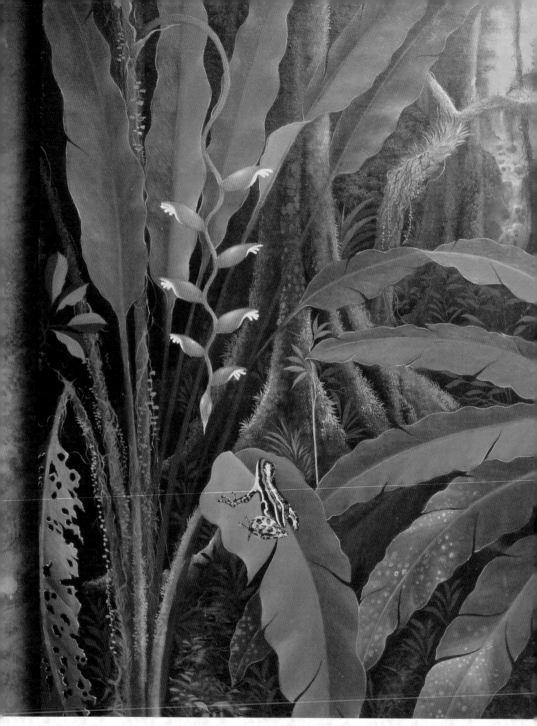

Heliconia flowers painted by Mauro Reategui Perez.
Perez is an artist from Pucallpa, Peru. He was born in a town on the banks of the
Ucayali River in 1973. A student of Pablo Amaringo, Perez is now an instructor at
the Usko-Ayar Amazonian School of Painting. Perez's paintings of flora, fauna, and
shamanistic tradition open a window into the extraordinary world of mind and spirit.
(www.mauroart.com)

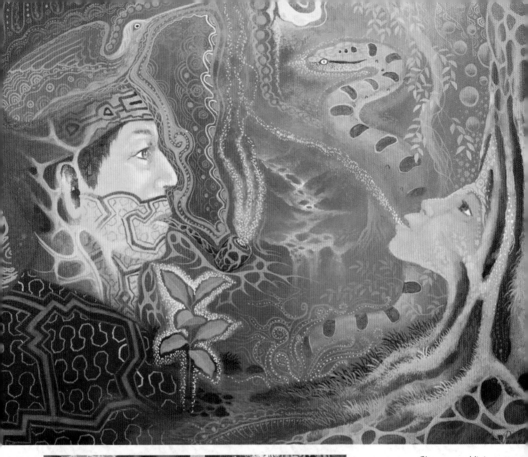

Chacruna Vision
by Mauro
Reategui Perez

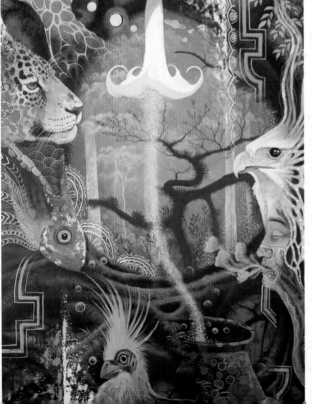

Pura Selva
by Mauro Reategui Perez

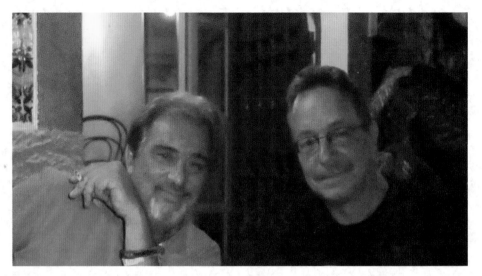

Investigative journalist Peter Gorman and author Alan Shoemaker
(photo by Raul Falch)

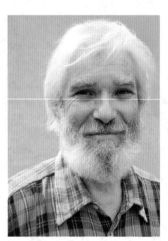

San Pedro shaman
Dr. Valentin Hampjes

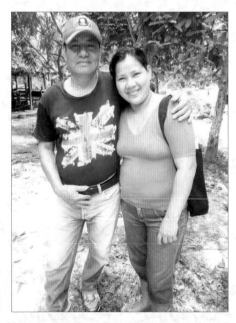

Ayahuasquero Don Juan
Tangoa and his wife,
Leonore

RETURN TO ECUADOR

During the next six months I moved from one healer to another, searching for one I felt could teach me. The quality of the ayahuasca always differed, and never was it as potent as the Siona healer's. Skepticism continually gnawed at me, preventing me from completely accepting as visions the many hallucinations I received in the fifty or sixty healing rituals I participated in and assisted at during that time. I failed to really secure my beliefs in the spiritual plane of existence that I thought I had seen so vividly on the banks of the Putumayo River. Yes, I was working with, speaking with, and witnessing many spirits, but I had difficulty completely believing that the plane of existence I was accessing was real. None of the curanderos I worked with seemed to be the one whom I felt I was destined to work with. Their singing of the icaros, in many cases, was too robotic, lacking the sensitivity I felt should naturally be there. Others I tested obviously just wanted money. Each of the various teachers I came to told me that he was the only true healer around, and anyone else I might decide to work with was just a brujo, an evil witch doctor. In many ways I appreciated this egotistical information, as it made my decision to move on easier, so that I could continue my search for my true teacher.

A little over a year after my experience with the Siona shaman, as I was preparing for a return trip to see Valentin in the mountains of Ecuador, I was informed of yet another curandero on the outskirts of Iquitos, Peru. I knew that one of the most precious gifts I could take to my maestro in Ecuador would be a bottle of freshly brewed ayahuasca, because the vine doesn't grow in the chill of the Andean high altitude.

I wandered through a small village, persistently asking directions from the locals for the house of their community curandero. All of the homes in the neighboring villages on the outskirts of Iquitos are built on very small plots of land. They usually don't have anything in the way of a garden, as over the years the land has been so washed with rainwater that growing a garden of any sort is out of the question for lack of nutrients in the soil. The houses are also plotted very close to one another. I finally rounded a corner at the back edge of a pueblo and came to a small, typically unpainted wooden-slatted, thatched-roof home. I called out, "Hello," and the door was opened by a young Peruvian girl who registered not the slightest bit of interest that a gringo was now standing before her. She called for her father. When he came into the house and our eyes met, I felt I was meeting a kindred soul. He was smiling inwardly and an air of humbleness issued from his body language. He walked me through his house to his backyard, which was full of various medicinal plants and four times as large as any other yard in the neighborhood. It even had grass growing in the center, which normally is machete-chopped out by the locals, who prefer bare clay and daily sweeping to keep it clean. I explained that I would like to take a bottle of ayahuasca to my San Pedro maestro in Ecuador and asked if he could provide me with one.

"Si. I can have it ready for you tomorrow." He took me to his own patch of ayahuasca vine he had planted on the back edges of his property. "You have a San Pedro maestro in Ecuador?"

"Si, Don Juan. I was working with San Pedro before I began working with ayahuasca."

"And you will be returning here to the jungle again?" he inquired as he finished chopping the vine.

We gathered the pieces and walked back to his home. As I shook his hand, we made plans to meet the next day, and he told me, "When you return from the mountains, you come back here. If you like, you may study here with me." This was the first time an ayahuasquero had invited me to apprentice. In the past I had visited the healers with this question in my mind. This time it issued naturally from him. The following day I returned to his home and paid him for his freshly cooked bottle of medicine.

When I arrived in Ecuador and presented the medicine to Valentin, he immediately asked me about the spiritual orientation of the man who had cooked it. His concern was not that the ingredients were correct or that the cooking had not been managed properly. Ayahuasca, after all, is a rather simple medicine to make. His interest was geared toward what types of energies the chef would have put into his pot. I could only confess that I did not know, but that the short time I had been around Don Juan the feelings I had for him were quite soulful. Valentin placed it in his refrigerator for safekeeping.

The following Friday, before we began the San Pedro ritual, I described the many ceremonies I had been involved in as well as a wide variety of curanderos and their various styles and belief systems. Valentin was concerned that I had compromised myself and had even picked up some bad energy while working with ayahuasca. He then proceeded to explain the meaning of this night's ceremony to the clients who had come:

"On a psychological level we have all been programmed by our peers, family, and society in general to behave in specific ways that have been deemed appropriate and acceptable. This includes most importantly those patterns ingrained so deeply that it is very difficult for us to change them. Our wisdom has outgrown most of the habitual emotional response patterns we have so meticulously developed, and now, in adulthood, we find ourselves burdened with an antiquated emotional language that we do not know how to rid ourselves of so that we may move forward into full realization. During this evening, with full realization through San Pedro, it is possible to focus your thoughts onto whatsoever psychological character traits you no longer desire and wrap them up, locking them away into the semblance of a safe deposit box, to which only you have the key, never to see or deal with them again unless you desire to do so. It puts you into the driver's seat, so to speak. The medicine will allow you, if you can singularly focus your thoughts on specific issues, to rid yourself of any and all manifestations you think are incongruent with your continued emotional growth. On a physical level the medicine will seek and destroy. As you drink the medicine you can literally feel it moving through your system, from the tips of your toes to the very crown of your head. As it is coursing through your body, it lingers here and there a bit longer, and it is in those areas that the medicine has found that you need more assistance."

He began the ceremony as usual, praying and blowing mapacho tobacco smoke and handing out shots of tobacco juice followed by San Pedro. When it became obvious we were beginning to feel its effects, he asked Mohita and his wife to take me into the back room to cleanse me of the negative energies he thought I had picked up in the jungle. Mohita had me lay face down on the massage table, removing jewelry and clothing. He sprayed me with agua florida and began sweeping me from head to foot with the shacapa. When he reached my thighs a look of shock came onto their faces, and I started to rise up, but Mohita stopped me, saying, "Don't get up, Alan, just stay here. We'll be right back." Twenty minutes later they returned, finished cleansing me, and I rejoined the others in the ceremony. The following morning I asked him what had happened.

"When I reached your legs, sweeping the shacapa over you, two tiny hands came out of your thighs. I continued sweeping at them but they were holding on. Finally a small man jumped out of your body and ran into the ceremonial space. We left you there to find him and chase him out."

"Did you find him?" I asked.

"No, we didn't. It is really of no importance. We call these *elementals*, and they don't do any harm."

Hearing their story didn't startle me, as interestingly enough this same small man had now reappeared for the third time in my life. The first time was when I was visiting my family for a weekend during my university days. I picked up some clay that belonged to my nephew and haphazardly began playing with it as I was watching television. When I looked down, my hands had formed the perfect image of an old man, complete with a hat and wrinkles in the pants. The next time the elfin man surfaced was when I was working on a movie called *Brubaker*, whose setting was a prison. One day following shooting, my friend and I returned to my sports car in the prison parking lot. There was a Polaroid camera in the rumble seat, and when my heavyset friend sat down in the passenger's seat, the camera fell to the floor and the flash went off. We watched the resulting photograph develop: a tiny man, again with hat and rumpled pants. I thought about this little man occurring three times in my life now. And my conclusion is that because I'm part-Irish, I've got my own little lucky leprechaun hanging with me.

As the sunlight slowly entered the room, I was very relaxed, lying on the couch directly across the room from the altar, which, being next to the door, receives the first soft light. Spacing out on the altar, tired and not thinking, my internal chatter was completely shut down, and it was at this point that I began to *see*. On the table and on the wall behind the altar I very calmly began noticing things moving. The image that appeared was an early morning landscape in the country-side, a mystical movie in 3-D. I observed the vision without giving it much thought for what must have been ten minutes until a bird flew from one perch point to another, for what must have been the third or fourth time. It was then that I realized that I was seeing into another reality or dimension. A voice began to speak to me, giving me the names of the trees, plants, birds . . . of everything that existed in this world on the altar. The vision continued for several minutes until everyone got up and headed outside to the backyard for the morning's sinus tobacco purge. Valentin asked if I was coming but quickly noticed that I was transfixed in deep space, staring at the altar. He gave me a knowing nod and continued on out. It was only then that I realized how long I must have been staring at the altar as the full light of the morning was upon us. Either my internal dialogue started up again, or perhaps it was the interruption, I simply don't know, but my visions stopped. It could have been that I was thinking too much; I was analyzing, intellectualizing. I wandered out to the back of the house, sat down next to Valentin, and explained what I had seen—that I had been seeing into another world that had manifested itself within the altar. He smiled at me and said, "The plant is finally showing itself to you, Alan."

After this experience I more and more began to look forward to each ceremony. Each time I drank the San Pedro, I had to ask Valentin to give me a larger dose, explaining that I was not here for healing, not here for homeopathic doses.

"Alan! Why do you want to drink so much?"

"As I explained to you before, Valentin, I am trying to break through a barrier. I am trying to *see*," I responded.

Eager for more interdimensional travel, I began spending every morning following the all-night prayers and chanting staring at the poster of the Virgin Mary above the door. One morning, as I was engrossed in her beauty, the image of the face of an old woman appeared, which quickly transformed into a skeleton. I was comfortable with the various expressions she would shift into from time to time, but this hallucination not only startled and confused me, it bewildered me. I went to Valentin, who was outside administering tobacco juice into the sinuses of the ceremony attendees, and told him what I had seen.

"You can see that in the face of María?" He was shocked. "Alan, you have picked up some very negative energy from the brujos in the jungle. How is it possible you have seen such ugliness in María?"

"No, Valentin. I have not picked up anything from the jungle. I *saw* it. I was simply hoping you might have an explanation for me."

"Alan, when you are in ceremony you must conduct yourself as a warrior. You must put forth sufficient energy that extraneous thoughts and energies cannot enter into your concentration. You must sing with more energy and not allow yourself to relax as much as you do."

My experience had led me to conclude that it was precisely a lack of focus that brought me closer to other realms of experience, but here was another point on which Valentin, a believer of Castaneda, and I diverged. Castaneda had been a graduate anthropology student at the University of California, Los Angeles. He and his wife would hold biweekly dinner parties and invite their fellow intellectuals. Each of the guests were to research some esoteric subject and make a presentation following dinner. Carlos apparently never made a presentation at these gatherings, but he certainly paid close attention to the others. For his university thesis he creatively combined many of these presentations into the now well-known story of how he had found a sorcerer named Don Juan Matus, who became his teacher. The thesis was accepted, and shortly afterward it was published and became a bestseller. Once the university officials discovered that the thesis had been fabricated, they were reluctant to expose Castaneda as a fraud because of the influx of new students applying to UCLA because they had read his number-one bestseller.

I had read Castaneda's books while tucked away in a private library in Quito. When I finally stuck my head out of that shell, I noticed that I had come out into the light with less respect for Castaneda's words than Valentin had. I noted many incongruences in the writings and simply could not accept what Castaneda was delivering as experiential studies in shamanism and sorcery. I discussed my thoughts about Castaneda with Valentin, but I couldn't seem to sway him over to my point of view.

During the next San Pedro ceremony I made an effort to expend more energy, giving Valentin the benefit of the doubt. When daylight broke, the group went outside, and Valentin began administering the tobacco juice into each person's sinuses. Just as they were finishing up, Madann, a good friend of Mohita's, arrived with his wife, an older woman of perhaps sixty-five years. She complained of having a sense of being full and was hoping Valentin might cure her. She drank a cup of tea and relaxed there in Valentin's living room with me.

"I feel much better now, thank you for the tea," she said. "I think I'll go to the small house and hold a women's prayer circle." And she left.

Later, I too went to the other house, and Valentin, Mohita, and I listened intently from an adjoining room as the women prayed together. Madann's wife was leading them in prayers to the Virgin María, holding a rosary in one hand and a Bible in the other. I listened for about twenty minutes, then returned to Valentin's house and relaxed while looking up at the poster of María again. After about fifteen minutes, the face of the woman leading the prayers of the Virgin superimposed itself on the face of María. She was smiling down at me with rosy cheeks, vibrant and healthy. It was a beautiful vision, and I wanted to leave and tell the woman leading the prayers what I had seen. At that moment, Valentin rushed into the room.

"Alan! Who is in this bathroom?"

"The young girl who had attempted suicide by drinking Drano. I've checked her—she's okay," I said.

"Then please grab the ax and hurry with me. The old woman must be in the other bathroom outside. She's not answering the door and I can't open it. Hurry, Alan!"

I grabbed the ax and wedged the door open. When I looked in, I saw the woman lying beside the door, eyes open but vacant. I squeezed into the room and took her pulse. She was gone. We carried her outside, and Valentin and I administered mouth-to-mouth resuscitation and heart massage. It was too late; she was dead. It was then that I realized that the vision of her I had received only moments earlier had occurred at the very moment she had died. That vision appeared again in my mind—the old woman as María, smiling down at me with rosy cheeks, a woman who had found her peace. We carried her into the medicinal room and laid her down onto the massage table. We lit candles and as all of us surrounded her, Valentin said prayers. While we were waiting for the ambulance to arrive, Madann decided he wanted to see her one last time. He returned to us in a state of shock.

"Valentin! Alan! Please come and look at her again. I think she's breathing!" We hurried into the room to check. Valentin was searching for a pulse and I tried to determine if she was breathing by placing a mirror under her nose. Finally, Valentin announced, "Of course she is dead. Alan had a vision of her as she passed through to the other side. She has certainly gone."

An autopsy was performed a few days later. She had died of a pulmonary embolism while straining to relieve her bowels. The sensation she had described of feeling full that morning was due to the embolism, which had exploded while she was straining on the toilet. She had literally drowned, falling to the floor. It occurred to me that I had predicted her death a week earlier without realizing it, as the earlier vision of an old woman transforming into a skeleton flashed in my mind. That morning, as she passed on, she had graced me with another.

I continued working with Valentin in many more ceremonies until I felt it was time to return again to the jungles of the Amazon and its medicine, ayahuasca. I informed Valentin of my decision to leave, and that I would be there on Friday for a final ritual. As always he was disturbed that I would be working with other teachers, but I sensed that I had more of an affinity for the jungle and ayahuasca than the Andes and San Pedro.

I arrived late on Friday evening. Valentin began the ceremony just after I arrived. As usual I asked him for two glasses of his medicine and, somewhat haughtily, he gave them to me. Two weeks earlier I had come across datura bushes in full flower and had given them to Valentin's assistant Mohita to dry and prepare for me. Mohita had been trained in datura by his maestro in Argentina and was prepared to introduce me into the mysteries of this quite dangerous plant. When Valentin had seen the flowers drying, he became distressed by the fact that I had an interest in working with this plant, as it is primarily used by the brujos for doing their ill-fated work.

As the ceremony began Valentin asked me to exchange seats with a woman who was sitting next to the altar, suggesting that the male and female energies would be better balanced if I did this. It was a strange request. In all the ceremonies I had participated in, Valentin had never arranged the room in any particular manner. But of course I did as he suggested. In doing so I would be the first person served the medicine. Valentin gave me the first glass, which was sitting on the altar, already full. It seemed a bit strange as he normally poured the medicine in front of us before we drank, but I drank it down anyway and, as usual, asked for another. After all, it would be my last ceremony with him, at least for a while.

It was a large gathering, perhaps twenty people, and it was the strongest San Pedro I had ever drunk. I clumsily made my way outside to purge about two hours into the ceremony and returned to my seat near Valentin and the altar. At one point I attempted to help Mohita and Valentin, who were working with a client on the massage table in the healing room, but as I walked into the room I moved through many spider webs of energy networks, or so it seemed, and there stood Mohita with Valentin. On the massage table was a beautiful young German woman whom we were going to work on. However, behind Valentin and Mohita were many other people—spirits of men and women, some dressed in doctor's attire. I simply didn't have the strength to deal with this at this time, so I returned to the security of my seat in the ceremonial room. I basically chickened out; I knew it. I just did not have the power and the will to continue.

About four hours into the ceremony Valentin began chanting the Lord's Prayer in Spanish, over and over, and the others in the room chimed in. When they had repeated this prayer maybe five times, I decided that I, too, would recite the Lord's Prayer, but I would chant it in English and for the express purpose of giving healing to Jamie, one of the attendees. Jamie had been coming to the ceremonies every week because he had what the Western doctors described as incurable kidney cancer. As I began chanting the others in the room chanted with me, but in Spanish, such that I thought that they enjoyed me doing this. So, I continued repeating the prayer, over and over. I must have done the prayer ten times until finally I was tired and thought I should let it rest for a while. Later in the morning they told me that they all thought I was going through some kind of hellish nightmare.

At first light I squinted my eyes and headed outside to Valentin's front yard. Calmly standing there on his normally manicured lawn were two large jungle cats of the size and appearance of jaguars, except that they were black with orange spots and surrounded by strange plants and vines. They were beautiful, and from the expressions on their faces they seemed to smile at me—they seemed to know me. I returned inside and told Valentin that someone had put something else in my San Pedro.

"Alan, why would someone put something in the San Pedro?"

"I don't know, Valentin, you tell me. All I know is that there were two very large black jungle cats surrounded by jungle waiting for me on your normally manicured lawn outside."

"I don't know what you're talking about, Alan."

Determined to get to the bottom of this, I returned outside and discussed the issue with Mohita. He told me that Valentin had seen the datura flowers drying and was very angry when he discovered they were for me. From this information, and the fact that Valentin had constantly warned me that I should be more careful about whom I drank ayahuasca with—that they could put other things in the medicine that I wouldn't be aware of until it was too late—I deduced that Valentin himself had played a cruel joke on me. I called Valentin outside to discuss my theory, and after a moment it became obvious that he had indeed doctored my medicine. I told him that he should never, ever put anything in the medicine that a person was not aware of or had not agreed to. In a rage I grabbed a handful of grass and threw it in his face and left the premises.

When I returned to Quito, I had an odd feeling that something was going to happen to me as soon as I arrived into Peru. I was in Sasha's apartment, bags packed and ready to be driven to the bus station.

Sasha said, "Alan, you seem preoccupied about something. Are you all right?"

"Yes, I'm okay. It's just that I have this feeling that as soon as I cross over the border into Peru something will happen to me. I can't tell what it is, but it is something I am not going to like. I have a feeling it is coming from Valentin, but I can't be sure."

I explained what had happened with Valentin as Sasha drove me to the bus station. Perhaps, I thought, if I spoke with Valentin before I left, I could dissipate the energy pattern that had been set up. I tried phoning him from the bus station but the lines were down. The sensation was becoming stronger and stronger, until Sasha suggested that I return to his home for the evening and delay my return to Peru until the next day. I agreed. I continued trying to phone Valentin but could not get through. The following morning, Sasha asked me if I still had the same feelings. "Yes, I do, but I don't think staying here will remedy anything. At least I am aware of it so that I can be on my guard." With that, Sasha drove me to the bus station, and from there I tried for the last time to phone Valentin. There was still no answer.

The bus ride to the border of Peru was about sixteen hours. I received my Ecuadorian exit stamp and Peruvian entry visa and hired a taxi to take me into Tumbes. My burro bag weighed in at over seventy pounds. Fortunately, the agency that sold me my onward bus ticket to Trujillo gladly allowed me to store it until the bus left. I wandered about the herb market in Tumbes, eventually purchasing four stalks of San Pedro and depositing them in my daypack. I still had two hours to wait until the bus left. Glancing around, I noticed a restaurant called Dos Hermanos (Two Brothers). I logically deciphered that this meant the uniting of North and South America, perhaps a symbol of the Incan prophecy of the eagle and condor, where all brothers of all races and all tribes will be united in peace; I decided that this would be a safe refuge until the bus left.

I found a table near an open window and sat down, placing my backpack, which contained my money and passport, on the table beside my cold beer so that I could keep an eye on it as I wrote in my journal. Shortly afterward, a couple passed by the window, and it seemed as though they were eyeing my pack. I realized someone could easily reach inside the window and grab it, so I moved it to a chair beside me and out of reach. If I could only get on the bus without anything happening to me, I felt I would make it out of this border town and avoid the terrible consequences I had sensed would come to me here. The same couple that had passed by the window returned and took a table across the room. I was getting paranoid as a result of their presence, but when the waiter arrived at their table I felt ridiculous. They both ordered a bowl of innocent soup. I must be fabricating this sense of doom because they obviously had not been looking at my daypack at all but had simply been looking for a place to eat. Perhaps they were even waiting for the same bus. I relaxed and continued writing in my journal. The workers in the restaurant cranked up the salsa, and all seemed right with the world. Twenty minutes later I turned to ask for my check. My pack was gone. The couple was gone. I ran outside, but they were nowhere in sight. Almost all of my money, my passport, and the San Pedro were gone, too.

I still had my bus ticket, so following a long, sad bus ride, I found myself in northern Peru, in Chiclayo, with four hours until the next bus left. I learned of a museum in the neighboring pueblo of Lambayeque and took a three-wheeled motor rickshaw there, beginning my very first tour of a South American museum. I traversed the first and second floors, taking in the various layouts of the old cultures and their art. Finally, I climbed the stairs up to the third floor, and as I rounded the corner I gasped in amazement: there before me, behind ten-foot-tall glass panels, stood a mannequin draped in a full-length robe of a checkered pattern. The colors had faded, but what interested me was the cut of the collar: Nerhu style. The sign below read: INCAN. This was original ancient Incan clothing! I had to sit down for a moment to fully integrate my thoughts, but then I absolutely knew for sure: the spirits I had seen back when I was on the Putumayo, who dressed in similar long checkered robes with a collar in Nerhu style, and those spirits that had been coming to me during my San Pedro and aya-huasca rituals, were not abstracts of a vivid imagination manifested by a potent psychotropic. They were real. My mind had not been playing tricks on me. I had not been hallucinating. I had never studied South American art or history, and so there was no way my visions could have been influenced by prior knowledge of the tribesmen that graced me with their visit in my visions on so many occasions. Here, standing before me, were their ghosts, appearing to me just as I had seen them before, but in the real, physical world. It took a moment for me to gather my thoughts. There were no more doubts—I finally felt that I could begin my apprenticeship with the plants in complete sincerity.

DON JOSE FATIMA

Continuing by bus back to Iquitos, Peru, I decided to visit Valentin's teacher, an old ayahuasquero named Don Jose Fatima, of Pucallpa, Peru. A traveling companion I had met along the way, Gina, had a specific medical problem she hoped he might divine a cure for: she was thirty-four and hadn't had a menstrual cycle for over thirteen years. All possible allopathic tests had been performed in France without arriving at either a cause or cure. Explaining this to Don Jose, he deferred to his wife, a curandera who was more of an expert on female maladies. She listened to my description of Gina's problem, then asked, "Can you give me a cigarette, Alan?" I handed her one. "I need three."

Don Jose Fatima closed the wooden window covers, darkening the room. His wife banded three cigarettes together to resemble a pan flute and lit them. She watched as the smoke swirled up slowly, turning them, twisting her wrist first one way, then another. An ash fell off and she studied it carefully. The cigarettes had burned down more than halfway, and as she looked back and forth to Gina, to the ashes, and to the smoke, she finally asked, "Do you have a friend named Sasha?" We had been staying in Quito, Ecuador, with a man named Sasha, and I told her so. "No, Alan, this isn't a man. It's a woman, a black woman from many years ago."

Gina thought for a moment, and finally her face lit up. "Yes! I had a friend named Sasha years ago in France, a woman, maybe fifteen years ago or more." The two women looked at each other in that telepathic way men are so often envious of.

"Si, señorita. This friend you had many years ago, Sasha, used to have the same problem you have now." There was a long pause again as the meaning slowly sank in. "But she doesn't have the problem anymore. You do. This woman has taken your birthing power away. You must get it back. You must go and see her to do this."

"Do you mean that this woman has menstruation now, and she didn't before? That she took this from me? On purpose? Is she some sort of witch?"

Don Jose's wife gazed deeply into her eyes and repeated, "You must go and see her."

A year later Gina returned to France and, strangely enough, received a letter from her old friend Sasha the day after her arrival: Sasha wanted to see her. Later, when I visited Gina in France, I asked her what had happened.

"Well," she hesitated, "I haven't been to see her."

After a long, pregnant pause, I asked, "Did you at least write her back?"

"No," she said.

"Gina, I don't think you really want your power back."

Back to that evening: Gina, Don Jose's apprentice, and I drank ayahuasca in his house, which was located in one of the slums outside of Pucallpa. Don Jose was about eighty years old and said he didn't drink ayahuasca anymore. "It isn't necessary," he said. Recently, he had had a prostate operation, and the forces involved in purging were too strenuous for his body. I was surprised later during the ritual to see that he was right. He did not need to drink ayahuasca to work during ceremony. As I observed him it became apparent that he could reach the state required to heal by using only his mind, a phenomenon that I now understand occurs with many older shamans who have many years of experience working with ayahuasca.

Don Jose sat on a short stool throughout the ceremony, and I sat on the concrete floor next to him. No patients had come, as we had decided to conduct the ceremony at the last minute. The apprentice began whistling icaros and everyone spoke in curiously subdued tones. His wife explained that we dared not risk singing the icaros aloud because of the late-night thieves; it could be dangerous if they discovered gringos were in the house, as they might want to rob us.

Don Jose sat staring at me the entire evening, occasionally asking me how I was doing, which I found slightly annoying as it interrupted my train of thought. As there were no locals present for healing, I felt I had an opportunity to explore some of the techniques used in searching for animal spirits and wanted to maintain my concentration. I had skimmed several books on shamanism while visiting the United States and one of the most popular subjects was animal spirits. Every time I glanced up at Don Jose, he was staring down at me. I assumed he was trying to determine how his former student, who was my San Pedro curandero maestro, was doing by studying me. I thought this rather humorous because I didn't know what I was doing. I had never been taught anything about animal spirits. I thought it interesting that, from one of the books I had read, you could find your animal spirit by closing your eyes and listening to drumming. How absurdly simple it all seemed. Even though there was no drumming, I decided to experiment. Two hours into the ritual I looked up and found myself face to face with what appeared to be a milky-white substance floating in space in front of me. After the initial surprise wore off, I studied it, trying not to get cross-eyed during the process. And then it appeared. The substance took shape. It was in the form of a coyote. "I see you there," I whispered, and it swooped back and appeared to enter the head of Don Jose.

When the ceremony came to a close we prepared our beds on the concrete floor, right alongside Don Jose's entire extended family. I was exhausted but could not get to sleep because of the internal chatter that would not be silenced. Thoughts about the next day's travel logistics banged around in my mind. And then a baby began crying. A bit agitated and annoyed, I put a stop to the mind chatter and began trying to soothe the baby in my mind. The crying stopped, which I found a little funny, and then the mind chatter began again. As the mind chatter began, the baby started crying again. I mentally soothed, and, oddly enough, the crying stopped again. *That's funny,* I thought to myself. *Experiment time.* I let the thoughts roll, mentally cruising the various travel options for the next day's journey . . . and the baby started crying again. I soothed my mind and it stopped. Too many coincidences. I repeated this over and over just to make sure, and sure enough the mental chatter was always accompanied by the baby's crying, and the mental soothing accompanied by silence. *Very strange,* I thought, before finally drifting off to sleep.

We stirred awake in the morning, and Don Jose said to me, "Alan, you were very concentrated last night. What were you doing?"

I felt ridiculous as I didn't know what I was doing, or if he had any knowledge of, or interest in, animal spirits. I explained that I had been looking for my animal spirits, and when he responded with, "And did you find any?" I knew he understood.

"No, I didn't, but I saw one of yours."

As I watched for his reaction, the entire family came around behind him, scrutinizing me.

Don Jose just smiled. "What was it?" he asked.

"A coyote," I said. And while he gently nodded his head in affirmation, his family was more ecstatic, responding, "Si! si!" and one of the younger children even clapped his hands.

DON FERNANDO'S BREW

After visiting Don Jose Fatima, we continued on down the Amazon to visit another curandero, Don Fernando, who had a camp five kilometers into the jungle at Requena, where he ran ayahuasca tourism programs. Gina had studied here for three months two years earlier, drinking ayahuasca and hoping, along with the other tourists, for visionary experiences. In all of her rituals with Fernando, however, she had yet to be gifted with anything resembling even a hallucination, let alone a vision, which didn't seem to bother her as she told me she found the experience "profoundly meditative and very cleansing."

While living in Iquitos I had heard he brewed an extremely strong ayahuasca, although a bit heavy on the vine, which contains Beta-carbolines, so I was looking forward to drinking with him. He had personally invited Gina and me to his camp.

Requena is a moderately sized but depressed mestizo community of maybe 700 people, ten hours up the Amazon from Iquitos by a slow river-bus. We spent the night with a local Peruvian family and the following afternoon walked with Don Fernando and his lover five kilometers into the jungle to his camp. During the walk Don Fernando entertained us with some of the more outlandish hallucinations the gringos have had in his rituals. He also explained how he believes it to be unsound to sing icaros memorized from another maestro in his ritual unless specifically asked to do so—his subtle way of telling me not to sing anything.

He had invited the local Requena villagers to drink with us, and eighteen people showed up. In the largest and most centrally located hut in his camp, we drank his brew, sitting around the inside perimeter walls, quietly listening to the icaros he quite beautifully blew into a pan flute, alternating with plucking a one-stringed, guitarlike instrument. He was absolutely an artist, an entertainer, and I was reminded more of theater than curanderismo. I drank two small glasses of La Purga, and the evening passed rather humorously, as most of the villagers fell asleep around four in the morning, after having purged with forces ranging from quietly ladylike fortissimos to manly tubas syncopating a marching beat. That evening, I listened to a full symphony of regurgitation in utter psychotropic darkness. It was a pleasant experience, with none of the seriousness normally found when people have come to be healed. For this, I appreciated the evening and Don Fernando, and so too did the villagers who knew him. At daybreak you could hear them joyously laughing and carrying on pleasant conversations while they bathed in the nearby stream.

Now we were four: Don Fernando and his lover, Gina, and myself. In his open-air kitchen we had a heavy, undercooked bean soup breakfast and exchanged thoughts about the previous evening's show. Gina and Don Fernando had a chance to catch up, as there had been no opportunity to speak with each other since she left his jungle refuge five months earlier.

Don Fernando had to return to Requena and invited us to stay at the camp if we wished. Just before he left he gave Gina a bottle of ayahuasca for our use that evening. He informed us of the two spirits continuously with him and those that guard his camp. This conversation came as a complete surprise. It seemed he was telling me this because he thought I might have perceived it during last night's show, or maybe I had heard some odd things about him while visiting other curanderos. I realized it could also be his way of insuring we treat his camp with respect after he left. He related a heartfelt story of how on one occasion he requested these spirits guarding his camp to help him prevent loggers from cutting on his property. When the company began chopping close to his land, two of the loggers apparently died in bizarre ways, which he claims were the direct result of his guardian spirits. He seemed sincerely depressed about this, as he had only wanted the logging stopped. He did not fathom the spirits would or could actually cause anyone's death. Shortly after the slow death of one logger from a debilitating disease, the cause of which the doctors could never quite determine, the second logger came uninvited to Don Fernando's home during a party. The man danced, had a few drinks, and left, without ever actually mentioning anything about the death of his friend. He was attempting to befriend Don Fernando. The man said in passing conversation that he simply worked for the logging company and had no authority as to where they were told to cut. In a subtle way this was either his attempt to ask for safety while not actively and consciously suggesting that a brujo could have had any influence on his friend's death, or he was denying the possibility that malevolent spiritual energies could have been responsible.

Don Fernando explained, "I am not in control of these spirits. They are indeed evil and for some reason incredibly protective of me. There was really nothing I could do to help him, even if these spirits were responsible."

This man also died a few months later in a strange accident involving a bulldozer. Don Fernando told me he was sad, but these events were out of his control. He seemed completely sincere as he related this story, but because it was so totally bizarre I was unsure as to exactly what he was trying to tell me. Was he insinuating he was a brujo? That he had spirits protecting his camp? That two spirits always remained with him? I easily accepted this, as I also have my own guardian spirits. I've felt them, been contacted by them, and my San Pedro maestro has even seen them during rituals. But I was somewhat skeptical that his spirits could actually kill.

He then explained how Gina should be careful with whom she drinks. He told us that it is possible for men to come to her in spirit form in an attempt to have sex, and that she must recognize this as a real event and prevent it through strong concentration.

That evening Gina and I each drank one large dose from the bottle he left with us and entered the large conference hut, placing a mattress in the center of the room. We made ourselves comfortable, curling up under two blankets. As darkness slowly approached, I began chanting, singing the icaros learned from my maestro Valentin. After an hour or so, the medicine was in full effect. Gina, who was sitting on the mattress to the right of and slightly behind me, began having a conversation. I stopped singing, as I thought she must be talking to me—after all, we were the only people there.

"What is it Gina? What do you want?"

"Just keep singing, Alan. I'm not talking with you."

"You're not talking to me? Then who are you talking to?"

"Alan," she chided, "to the other people here from the village drinking with us."

"Other people from the village?" I asked. "How many other people are here, Gina?"

"Oh, I don't know exactly, but I'd say about twenty. Just look around for yourself."

But there were no other people. I knew what she must be seeing and explained that they were spirits of people, not flesh and blood. She just laughed it off. "Alan, will you please stop joking with me?"

She started walking around the large open space, making gestures as though she were going through invisible doors and entering rooms that weren't there. She began, quite pleasantly as a matter of fact, carrying on two- and more-sided conversations with people who weren't there, until she finally reached the darkest corner of the large room and began having a very long talk with what I now began to see as well were two people, one of whom was in a long, hooded black cloak.

I caught a glimpse of his face and noticed that it was milky white in color. Concerned, I thought that quite possibly there was a skeletal head under that black hood, as I couldn't help but associate negative forces with black clothing. I had no choice. I had to act as though this were a dangerous situation—especially after the breakfast conversation I had had with Don Fernando. I told Gina to return to the mattress immediately.

"Sit down here with me, please," I requested.

"I'd like to sit down with you awhile, but you have," and she counted them, "one, two, three . . . eight other people on the mattress with you. There simply is not any room, Alan," she rather pleasantly stated.

Finally I demanded that she sit down with me, and obviously to appease me she sat down on the mattress. As she made a place for herself next to me, I asked about the "friends" she had been speaking with in the corner of the room. "Yes, there are two of them," as I had seen. When I asked her to describe them to me, she did, but she didn't mention anything about a skeletal face. The clothing, however, was identical to my description. We were seeing the same thing. But as to their capacity for evil? It was better to be safe than sorry, especially after having heard the story told to me by Don Fernando.

"Gina, please listen to me. I see the same people, but you have to realize these are not of flesh and blood; they are spirits. And those two in the corner you have been speaking with? They are evil. Do you understand? I'm going to tell them to leave and you cannot go back over into that corner anymore, all right?"

She had such a wide-eyed, innocent expression on her face. Her whole demeanor was childlike, so I spoke to her as such.

"Okay," she said.

I rose from the mattress and nervously walked over to the dark corner. I had no idea what I was going to do, but as I got closer, a natural instinct came over me. With a strong hand gesture and a loud yell of "Vaya!" I demanded they leave. I no longer saw them, so apparently they got the message. I returned to the mattress and kept a close eye on Gina as I continued singing icaros.

But she couldn't sit still. I watched as she again began wandering around the room, opening many different nonexistent doors, working her way through a maze of rooms that weren't there. Finally she came back to me. Her behavior was strange, like a wild-eyed child's first visit to Disneyland. I was beginning to lose patience with her.

"Alan, would you like something to eat? They've made some food for us. It's hot."

"There's no food here," I said bluntly.

And like a silly little girl she said, "Of course there is, they just made it. It's ready!"

"Okay, bring me some."

I had hoped her actually trying to deliver food would help jolt her back to reality. She returned to the mattress without food, of course, and extremely confused. She described the kitchen, the very kind woman inside who handed her the tray of steaming food, but as she reached out to grab it, her hands went right through the tray. She couldn't understand what was going on. I explained again that these were spirits, not actual people, but she was completely incapable of comprehending this. The look on her face was one of utter confusion—a little scared, but mostly sad, as she felt she was somehow being manipulated by her new friends in a cruel joke.

"Alan, there are some more of my friends outside. It's raining and cold. Can I open the door and let them come in?"

"No, you cannot."

"I have one friend whose father is on the way to pick her up. Can she at least come in?"

"No. You cannot let anyone else in this room."

"Can I go to the bathroom?"

Ayahuasca typically purges you from both ends, neither of which we had done yet, so I lit a makeshift oil lamp, the base of which was a small coffee can with a wick coming out through a hole punched in the aluminum lid, and led her outside, down the ramp running over the shallow lake formed by the overflowing creek, and finally to the outdoor john. Then we began the return trip. Upon arrival, I held the door open for Gina to enter and looked back for her but she had disappeared into the absolute darkness of the moonless, overcast night.

"Gina!" I yelled.

"Yes?" She was only ten yards away but on a ramp at the edge of the deepest pool here.

"What are you doing?"

"This man here wanted me to talk to him for just a moment," she said.

"No, come here, right now!" and she did, immediately. Finally she listened and gave me, rather than the spirits, credence. Had she not, I don't know what would have happened. Perhaps she would have wandered off and drowned, or been led deep into the jungle in the middle of the night, a very dangerous place to be at that time.

Around four in the morning we decided to go upstairs and try to get some sleep. Just as I climbed inside the mosquito net, she saw something else.

"I'm sorry to bother you again, but could you tell that man to go away? He scares me and I don't like him."

This was the first time she had mentioned being scared the entire evening. She described a very large man with armbands and a loincloth with a bow drawn back, his arrow aimed at us. She was scared and I was too. I knew spirits could be more than just simple hallucinations, and even if these were hallucinations, the psychological damage they could cause could be long lasting. I commanded the spirit to leave, using the Spanish *Vaya!* I didn't know what else to do.

"Is he still there?" I asked.

"No. He's gone," she replied.

The entire night I completely believed, accepted, and responded to her visions and what she saw. There didn't seem to be any other way around it. I witnessed her maneuvering in and out of a maze of rooms all night. I watched and listened to her speaking and interacting with people who weren't there. I wanted to protect her, but I was unsure I knew enough to be of any real help. I only hoped that during the night, as I kept singing the icaros, we would be protected, and I feared that if this wasn't enough we could be lost; we could be in way over our heads and in some kind of trouble that, at the time, I really could not fathom.

Crawling back under the mosquito net we half-attempted to get some sleep, but it just wasn't possible. We returned downstairs as the dim light of the sun began filtering itself into the space, apparently sending the ghouls away and bringing Gina enough lucidity that she began to understand what had happened but was concerned she wouldn't completely come back. I sat again on the mattress in the center of the room, and she milled about the space, taking in the views of the jungle while the sun's light continued to bring her increased clarity. Then, in full daylight, she walked over to me and, in shock, told me she saw two very old women under the blanket with me. She wasn't as lost as she had been because the brew had worked its way through her system, but there was still enough residual in her body that she continued to have access to this other world, even in broad daylight. She was now aware enough to comprehend that these were spirits, and that she was capable of continuing to see into their reality. Slowly and steadily, as the morning progressed, she came around. Somewhere around noon we hiked the five kilometers back into sanity—to the Amazon River and Requena.

I believe that were it not for her strength of character, she could have suffered irreversible psychological damage from this bizarre experience. We spent the entire day talking about it, recalling all the events that occurred during the night, which helped her to process the overall experience. In so doing, with her maintaining complete lucidity without paranoia, she felt as though she became whole again.

Two weeks passed before I was able to ask Don Fernando about his brew. I questioned him about his use of datura and how much he had put into this batch. He insisted that its strength was due to the type of ayahuasca vine. He said it was negro ayahuasca and chacruna and had no datura in it at all. I realize that among the some 4,500 curanderos here in this region of Peruvian jungle called Loreto, there are many secrets, especially when it comes to their medicine. This drink, however, was not what I would call a medicine. There was obviously something else stirred into it besides *Banisteriopsis caapi* and *Psychotria viridis*. As far as I know, the addition of a negro ayahuasca, which is supposedly a much stronger type of ayahuasca vine, would only account for the presence of more harmaline and harmala, not more DMT, which is a psychedelic compound of the tryptamine family. The Beta-carbolines in the ayahausca vine increase your serotonin levels. This is why, years ago when *bipolar* was called *manic-depressive,* Beta-carbolines were prescribed by doctors to those having these problems. The half-life of DMT in your system is a maximum of four hours. Our ritual had begun at 6:00 p.m. and ended at 6:00 a.m., twelve hours later; I knew I would never get it out of Don Fernando exactly what it was he had added to his brew. I was reminded of the advice given by Valentin when I left for the Putumayo: "Be careful with whom you drink and certainly never drink more than they do."

When drinking alone, without the presence of a curandero, especially without the presence of the curandero who made the medicine and to whom the ritual space belongs, you must take it upon yourself to prepare the space. In North America the medicine men use the smoke from sage to clean the energies. In South America the typical method is to burn palo santo, "holy wood." Mapacho tobacco also works. This not only prepares the space by clearing out whatever spirits may be "nesting" there, but helps to put you in the correct psychological state by virtue of having gone through these steps. I knew these things when we drank Don Fernando's brew. I simply neglected to implement them. Just as a mother cautions the child about speaking with strangers, beware of drinking brews from those whom you don't know. Sometimes rule breaking can be dangerous.

THE POWER OF THE ICAROS

Just over five hundred years ago the Western world all but destroyed the great nations of the Americas. They could not have succeeded with the force of arms alone, so for some ungodly reason disease and fear spoiled cultures that would have been magnificent. And now a new era has begun. The desire to reassemble the pieces of the puzzle that may still be found, that we might somehow catch a glimpse of what was, and what still could be, haunts us. The most mysterious and precious of these pieces is the healer, or curandero. Embodied within their ancient form of healing is knowledge of mysticism and plant spirit medicine that may never be understood by modern, scientifically based medicine.

There exists a wealth of literature available on mysticism, shamanism, sorcery, magic, witchcraft, and so forth, dealing generally with personal experience and even giving rather precise instructions on how to find the various locations, teachers, and even the exact formulas necessary to turn a Sacred Power Plant into an entheogen. This ease of access to the mystical entheogenic formulas is startling and possibly dangerous. Taking any form of mind-altering medicine without preliminary rudimentary education and controlled investigation can lead to possible possession of the body by unknown subtle energies, permanent psychotic mental states, and even to a loss of the soul.

When under the influence of Sacred Power Plants, you leave yourself open to being possessed, which can be very dangerous, but more importantly, you hope the plant will show itself to you, enabling you

75

to understand its power and apprehend its uses as a medicine for healing. As the term *Sacred Power Plant* suggests, they are to be ingested with the intention of being taught medicine and healing capabilities by energies of the Light and the spirits of the plants.

As fascinating as accounts of otherworldly visionary experiences found in various books and magazines may seem, it is without a doubt something that should not be taken lightly. Negative energies and spirits can attach themselves to you and be extremely difficult to remove, even with the help of a curandero. Many people like to play shaman, but it is important to realize that simply having memorized the various icaros and singing them during makeshift rituals is not sufficient, and could even create more havoc by giving you a false sense of security. The vibrations set up from chanting icaros must come from a spiritual center within yourself, with such purity of purpose that your essence exudes the Light. I would also suggest that if you choose to play shaman, you do it in the presence of your maestro shaman, a true healer who has learned most of his icaros from the plants themselves.

In anthropologist Luis Eduardo Luna's scholarly work *Vegetalismo: Shamanism among the Mestizo Population of the Peruvian Amazon,* he writes, "The word *icaro* seems to be a loan word from the Quechua verb *ikaray,* which means 'to blow smoke' in order to heal. This term is used in various parts of the Peruvian Amazon among the mestizo as well as among ethnic groups of the Ucayali. The vegetalistas of Iquitos and other areas of the Peruvian Amazon also use the verb *icarar,* which means to sing or whistle an *icaro* over a person, an object, or a preparation to give it power.

The magic melodies known as *icaros* are usually taught to the curandero while he is under the influence of one of the many entheogenic Sacred Power Plants. The spirits of the plants literally present themselves to the curandero and teach him healing and blessing songs, both the melody and the words. The spirits also inform the curandero as to the particular purpose of the song—whether it is to be used for luck, love, soul loss, physical healing, or even to control and enhance the visions being received. There are thousands of icaros, and there seems to be a competition among the curanderos as to who has memorized the most. Some even believe that the more songs one knows, the more power you have, even when most of one's songs have come from apprenticing with various maestros. I have seen curanderos visit other healers' rituals undercover, just to steal that healer's icaros.

Icaros can come to you in your dream state as well as during a ritual. When in the dream state your vision is not blurred by events in your waking reality; your mind is more at ease and the ego is out of the way. Whether you are gifted from the spirits with an icaro when you are in your waking state or in your dreams, one thing seems to be a constant: you remember the icaro without it having to be repeated over and over. The languages that come with an icaro can be incredibly complicated and can contain more than one tongue.

When the old Siona ayahuasquero on the Putumayo gave me his harmonica, I immediately began playing the icaro I had heard him performing during his ritual. He listened intently as I repeatedly played it until he realized I had the basic tune. Then he stopped me, explaining that the secret was more in the vibratory pattern than in the melody itself. Again I played it repeatedly until he assured me I was getting the concept.

I have been told by my ayahuasca maestro not to overly concern myself with trying to memorize the words of an icaro, as being able to sing it from the heart, with the correct resonance and vibration, is more important. The icaros of the maestro curanderos are quite difficult to learn because in most cases there is a mixture of more than one language within the same song. An icaro might contain Quechua, Spanish, and any of a variety of indigenous tongues. One of my teachers even informed me that he had purposefully made some of his icaros almost impossible to memorize because he had many icaros that had been stolen by hungry curanderos visiting his rituals in disguise. It is out of respect to your maestro that you learn his icaros and eventually cant them for him.

During an apprenticeship you are usually required to air whistle the melodies of your maestro as he is singing. This shows him not only that you are paying attention, but that you are also giving him the proper respect when he is working. You may also softly sing the icaros with him, but never so loud that you overpower his voice. Remember, being able to mechanically recite the maestro's icaros does not a Mozart make. But how else are you to be taught? There may come a time when you begin gaining access to the spirits of the plants yourself and thus given your own icaros.

Icaros hold strong power, and their force is only for you. Many tribal healers call forth the young men of the community when they reach the age of twelve or so, to drink ayahuasca or another Sacred Power Plant. The following morning the curandero questions each boy about his visions the previous night. It is the child who tells of having seen the spirits of the plants that the curandero keeps and teaches; only a few of these boys will be able to withstand the sacrifices involved in the years of apprenticeship that ultimately make the curandero. Many young men fall into the ways of the brujo, a much easier path than that of the true healer.

Again, your true icaros come directly from the spirits of the plants. These are the basis of any healing power. You must, however, suffice yourself with the icaros of your teacher until such time as the spirits of the plants decide it is time to teach you, for ultimately your real teacher is not the curandero, it is the spirits of the plants. When they decide they like you, they will be by your side forever, and they will never let you down. You must learn to work with them and, as Valentin once told me, you must expend more energy in the chants and singing during the night to be strong. You cannot simply take these medicines and watch things happen. You must be an active participant, a warrior in maintaining the strength of goodness in your visions. If you do not, negative forces, influences, effects, and hallucinations can insert themselves into your consciousness.

If you memorize an icaro you have learned from a curandero, you may only be reciting, and so its power may also reflect that. It is, however, a beginning and shouldn't prevent you from continuing your studies. Good teachers are difficult to come by, so you must center your energy such that when you cant these icaros, the soul you expose is pure, humble, forgiving, gracious, endearing, egoless, and respectful of both the icaro itself and the maestro from whom it came. Ideally, your icaros should be learned from the spirits of the plants. However, only they decide when, where, and if you will be granted this gift. This power comes only to those who have been shown the path. The desire to become a healer isn't enough; you must have been granted this gift in order to properly pursue it. It is possible that the granting can come after the student has already been studying, as the spirits of the plants can decide to teach you at any moment. The power to convey the Light through the chantings comes from your soul being the plant's conduit. The purer you are spiritually, and the "cleaner" you are physically, the more powerful the incantations and their protection and more the likelihood of your being used by the energies of goodness. For let there be no doubt: There are at least two forces of spirits at work here. At least two.

DON JUAN TANGOA, AYAHUASQUERO

Looking toward the jungle always makes me smile. It is a coming home. As much as I liked Quito and my friends there, I kept yearning for the "green hell," as my ayahuasca maestro would put it. With the Amazon and the smaller tributaries snaking their way around below me and the green expanse extending forever, I get the sense of pulling a warm blanket up over my nose. Iquitos, Peru: I was back, and it was good to be home.

On my first day back I met a woman named Laura, a gringa from Holland who had just opened her arts-and-crafts shop smack in the center of the tourist district. Things were nicely laid out in the shop, with various things from both the jungle and the Andes. She was doing well and had recently moved into the home of a curandero who lived outside of Iquitos who was her maestro, she told me. She appreciated the comfort and security of living with a family, especially one that had an ayahuasquero, as she was looking for emotional healing. The following morning, after hearing many great things about this man, I decided to visit his home in the hope of meeting him, and as it happened he turned out to be the same curandero from whom I had received a half-gallon of ayahuasca to be taken to Valentin on my last trip to Iquitos. At that time he had suggested that when I return from Quito I come and study with him. Now Laura was there, too.

Don Juan Tangoa, ayahuasquero, was his name. He was a healer and specialist who worked with ayahuasca. He had been drinking ayahuasca since he was thirteen years old. He was only forty-three at the time, which is very young for a curandero, but you could see from the look in his eyes that he was a gifted man. We arranged a ritual for three nights later.

I arrived at Don Juan's escorted by Laura. He had built a small shed beside his jungle-style home, which he used for ayahuasca ceremonies. His home was simply made, with inexpensive wood, a leaf-thatched roof, and dirt floors. It was located in a part of town that was close to the airport. Laura told me that Don Juan had never taken on an official apprentice before and that for him to offer this to me was rather unusual. He had attempted to teach apprentices in the past, she said, but the men he had tried to teach quickly became competitive with him and he had given up after a short while.

Don Juan came out of his house to join us. He was a handsome man, in good physical condition, and had vibrant, smiling light coming from his eyes. He told me to always sit on his right when we were together in ceremony. This chair was reserved for his apprentice. I would be the first to drink, and if he had to consult with me I would be there so we could speak quietly to each other. He especially enjoyed talking about his days in Cambodia when he, along with other Peruvian jungle fighters, had been hired to go in and help liberate any U.S. prisoners after the Vietnam War had ended. He had been shot twice while playing the mercenary and that is how he came to know Philadelphia, or at least the hospital there, where he recuperated until they sent him back to Peru. He never received payment for this work, and it had embittered him toward the States. *Join the club,* I thought.

I sat beside Don Juan, and Laura sat on her camping mattress beside the door. Don Juan explained to me that her seat was an important placement during the ceremony; it is essential to have this area safeguarded so that malevolent energies won't enter the space. The only other accoutrement was a white towel that he placed around his shoulders. Before he began the ceremony he placed it over his head with only his face exposed, which gave him a saintlike appearance. Laura told me that it is standard to purchase a pack of cigarettes for curanderos prior to every ceremony, and I had done that—one pack of Lucky Strikes. While the local tobacco was chemical free and I had many pouches of American Spirit tobacco, he preferred the smoother, prepackaged gringo cigarettes. He began to bless one of the cigarettes by air-blowing an icaro into it and then lit it up and began blowing smoke into the half-gallon container that held the ayahuasca.

This ceremony was special. The community hadn't been informed about it, so nobody else had come in for healing. It was to find out whether or not he and I could work together. He asked me some questions to determine how much experience I had and then poured my cup to the brim. I drank it down quickly and hoped his medicine would be of the potency I desired because it tasted so terrible I would hate to have to drink another cup. Laura followed, and then Don Juan drank.

Don Juan had the demeanor of a healer, a true shaman. He was obviously a very spiritual man. He was here to heal, treating locals in his community and people who came from far-off communities who were suffering from illnesses that they had no cure for. If they had money to pay for healing, fine. If they had a chicken to trade, that too was okay. If they had nothing, he would do what he could for them as well. Impressive.

As we sat there waiting for the ayahuasca to take effect, he began singing, and this immediately caught my full attention. Don Juan had a honey-smooth voice, and his mastery of the icaros was impressive. He continued singing, one after another, occasionally lighting another cigarette between icaros. He made me feel very comfortable in my choice of my new maestro.

The next morning we discussed what he required of an apprentice: acceptance of his tactics and belief system without question; preparation of the space for each ceremony; helping with the cooking of the ayahuasca and acquiring the necessary ingredients in order to do so;

absolute loyalty; and no drinking with other curanderos or discussing his particular secrets about his brews or his methods of healing with anyone other than him. He also insisted that I follow his dietary requirements to the letter, which included abstinence from sex for a minimum of four days before and following each ritual. I would be required to quietly air whistle the icaros he sung during ceremony to demonstrate that I was paying attention and attempting to learn and memorize the icaros, never falling asleep during ceremony, concentrating at all times on the healing issues at hand, and generally being around when he needed me.

This was just what I had wanted—definite rules. I told Don Juan that I liked the ayahuasca strong, and he suggested that I drink as much as I wanted. This contrasted with Valentin, who wanted me to drink no more than he did. It was then that I knew I could work with Don Juan. He was a very serious healer and also a very charming man, an essential ingredient to being a successful curandero. He would never ask for money and I knew that. The subject was never brought up. In the days to come I would pay my share, however, buying food for the children and family while I lived there.

I moved in with Don Juan and his family a few days later. The space was very cramped, and at night the only privacy I had was a simple mosquito net that was pulled down around my bed. The home consisted of two rooms: the kitchen and the bedroom. In the bedroom were four beds, and doubling up was normal: Don Juan and his wife, Leonore, with her first child, Gabiche, in their bed; his oldest daughter (from his first, and late, wife), Consuela, and her two-year-old child, with her younger sister, Rosillo, in another bed; and Willy, Don Juan's son, and his cousin in another bed. The clothes were hung from sixteen penny nails hammered into the planks making up the walls of the hut. Two dogs with a fresh litter of pups lived outside, along with twenty chickens, two turkeys, two pigs, and his fighting roosters. Needless to say, it was a tight space for such a large family, but no one seemed to think twice about it. This was going to be home for me now, and I was taken in as family from the first day I arrived.

The family quickly learned my name, and the women became accustomed to adding my dirty clothing to the bundles they hand-washed on a daily basis. It was a happy family and laughter was often heard from the time I woke up in the morning till everyone pulled their mosquito nets down around them at night. We woke up every morning at sunrise, roosters crowing, and opened the window to let in the sunlight. It was fascinating to see the family watching TV on the old black and white tube. I loved listening to the laughter of Consuelo, Juan's oldest daughter, which was light and easy. She had a pleasant attitude, which was nice to see in a young woman who was only sixteen years old and already had a son two years of age. She had lost an eye to childhood pranks when her brother, Willy, stuck a pencil in her eye. That had been years ago, and she had adjusted. She was beautiful, and the wandering eye did little to affect her. If anything it only made her appear a little spacey until you knew why.

It was here, on the dirt-floored kitchen, that I was introduced to the delicacies of *caiman* (crocodile) and monkey soup. Fresh caiman was my favorite. It tasted somewhat like a mix of chicken and lobster, but leaning to the lobster side. Monkey was also delicious. These animals had been wild and were hunted, not for their skins or to sell to tourists, but so the family could eat. Usually the meat was brought to Don Juan as payment for healings he had done. It is important to trade something or give back when you come for healing; it helps you to open up to receive the medicine, an essential part of the healing process (for more on this subject, see appendix 2).

Don Juan and I held ceremony every Tuesday and Friday night. He loved singing his magical icaros, and of all the different curanderos I had participated in ceremony with, Don Juan surpassed anything I had heard before. I felt very blessed to have found my maestro and was looking forward to learning more about the path of the ayahuasquero.

I would continue my studies with him for over two years. It was here that I had my first two experiences in healing, as well as my own initiation as a curandero-ayahuasquero.

Don Juan always made himself available to those seeking a cure. I was always amazed at the types of illnesses we would encounter at his ceremonies. Most often the curing would be based around a sickness, or *daño,* that was caused through the actions of a brujo. Don Juan would sing icaros designed specifically to counter the effects of this *brujeria,* or black magic. He often would place his right hand on the affected area in order to pull out the illness, normally caused by either a *virote,* which is an interdimensional magical dart shot into its intended victim by a brujo or from an evil incantation. Another means of effectively countering the effects of brujeria is with tobacco smoke and the use of the shacapa.

Don Juan was always careful as to which patients he would accept, for if one of them were to die on his property it would put him in danger with the Peruvian authorities. We did, however, decide to take one patient who later passed on two months after returning to her home. While she was still alive her husband had carried her to Don Juan and laid her down on a bamboo mat in the center of his dirt-floored ritual hut.

"Alan, please take a look at this woman and tell me what you think." He asked me to raise her blouse and look at her stomach. Floating there in her stomach cavity was a large object, foreign to the body.

"Place your hand on it Alan," he told me. Placing my hand just above her belly button, I felt what seemed like a petrified object, rock-hard and cratered, about the size of a grapefruit.

"Come outside and talk to me," he then said.

I told Don Juan that in my opinion this woman should be sent to the hospital. He quietly informed me that she had already been there and they had sent her away, telling her they could find nothing. Her husband told me that the three times he had previously taken her to the hospital, the ball in evidence before us now was hidden, and the X-rays showed no evidence of any abnormality. That was difficult to believe.

We decided to work with her and arranged for her to stay on a cot in the ceremonial space. Within the first week the ball disappeared somewhere into her stomach cavity. Then her left leg, from the top of her thigh to her knee, began to swell up like a balloon. The pain was agonizing for her and was only somewhat relieved when I massaged her lower back around the spine, something I did on a daily basis. At times it became so intense that I purchased pain medication from the Iquitos pharmacy for her. Don Juan continued making various herbal drinks for her, and we continued performing ayahuasca ceremonies for four weeks in her presence, without any effect. She was not served. She lost weight and the pain and swelling increased.

In desperation, we finally decided that perhaps she should drink ayahuasca herself, and so we conducted a ritual. After the effects of the ayahuasca set in, Don Juan asked me to try to see what was causing the problem, using a curandero's x-ray-like vision. I tried looking into her body but nothing came. Don Juan was determined that this situation was caused by a brujo and that he held enough power to reverse it. Curanderos are careful to accept only those cases of brujeria they believe are caused by a brujo weaker than they are. Finally, a message came to me, perhaps more out of my own frustration with the situation than from any actual vision. Even now I'm not sure. Don Juan, who was as frustrated as I was, was demanding that a healing come forth. I felt so helpless. I remember thinking that even if I get no clear vision of the cause of the problem, that perhaps I should fabricate something just for their sake. The power of the mind and the placebo effect came into my thoughts as I told him, "Don Juan, I see a two-headed snake that has moved from the lower stomach down into her left leg. It can't maneuver past the knee joint and it can't turn around—that's why we have all the swelling. The rock-hard ball that we saw floating in her stomach a month ago is its feces sack, which is being pulled along behind it."

This was quite a fantastic synopsis, especially since I wasn't sure exactly how I had come to this conclusion. Intuition is one thing, and clairaudience is another, yet it is still difficult to distinguish the difference. That ability comes only through years of experience. Don Juan called me outside the ritual hut to discuss our next move.

"Good. A two-headed snake. Are you absolutely sure?" he asked me.

"Well, I don't know, Don Juan. But that's what I feel."

I knew I was giving him the type of information that he needed so he could at least begin working on a specific cure. I also felt that I had fabricated this out of a sense of sympathy for both Don Juan and the woman. Truth be told, I was confused.

"Listen to me," he said. "I will sing an icaro of a bird that normally eats snakes. With this icaro I hope to invoke its spirit into the ritual to eat the snake she has inside of her. This is a difficult thing to do, so I must concentrate very deeply. You can help me by watching for the bird. Let me know when you see it."

Now I felt that I could be getting us even deeper into a black hole. In my attempt to alleviate the anxiety of Don Juan and the woman, I unwittingly might only heighten their frustration if no healing were to come about. What a mess I had created.

We returned to the ritual. Don Juan started singing this icaro repeatedly, but I saw nothing. Finally he moved over to the woman and began trying to pull the snake out using a cupping motion of his hand on her lower thigh. Again I saw nothing. He kept asking me, on each of his attempts to draw the snake out, and I continued to tell him, "No. Nada, Don Juan." I realized that because I had gotten us into this situation with my so-called seeing, that perhaps it would be best to tell him that I was beginning to see things leaving her leg while he frantically attempted to remove the energies. As I did so I could feel a change in the energy of the room. It was almost as if I could hear an audible sigh of relief, not only from Don Juan, but from the woman as well.

The next morning, when I went to check on the old woman, she had noticeably changed. She was relieved, and there was substantially less pain. In the next few days she decided the time had come to return home to her family. When her husband arrived to get her she was able to walk out on her own accord. We were pleased that she left his home in better condition than when she first came to us but realized that a complete healing did not come about.

Don Juan sadly informed me that the brujo who had inserted this illness into her was stronger than he was. Two months later her husband saw me in Iquitos and informed me that she had passed away. While I still felt that the snake was pure fabrication, I also understood very clearly how, under certain circumstances, it was important to give the patient (and sometimes even the healer) something to believe in, for I knew that the healing powers inherent in people, when activated, could absolutely cure anything. Don Juan believes this as well and often works in this way, which reinforced my belief that the image of the two-headed snake was real, regardless of my doubts. I felt that under the circumstances he could not have come to any other conclusion himself.

A few months later Don Juan's wife, Leonore, was bitten by something on the pulse point of her left wrist. She came to me in frustration. The tiny bite was continually itching. It looked like nothing more than a small mosquito bite. After a week's time, this very small bite transformed into a volcano rising up out of her wrist, the height of my small fingernail, with a diameter of about one inch, oozing creamy-white pus. Don Juan and I were baffled. I asked the military doctors in Iquitos what their opinion was, but they too were perplexed. They suggested that we pour powdered penicillin directly into the open wound.

I tried this, and the fever that Leonore had begun to suffer from subsided for two days, but the wound continued growing and seeping pus.

We watched helplessly as large knots of some sort of cartilage-type material began forming, starting first on her wrist around the bite, and then moving up her arm about two inches every day until it reached her shoulder. Leonore's left arm was as hard as a rock, and the volcano continued growing in size as her fever returned full force. When these hard knots began moving down into her chest, possibly moving toward her heart, I sought in vain for some relief for her from the military doctors. The following morning, Don Juan came to me in desperation, suggesting we drink ayahuasca that evening in the hope of divining a cure.

"Si, Don Juan, of course," I agreed rather nervously. It seemed that when he presented me with this idea he was asking me to divine the cause of her illness, a responsibility I felt both reluctant to accept and incapable of handling. Immediately, we began to prepare the medicine.

Don Juan cut vines that he had grown on his half-acre property, and I searched for chacruna, the admixture plant necessary to produce an entheogenic state. He had only the very small plants I had gifted him growing there on his property. When I returned from purchasing some chacruna from the local Iquitos plant market in Belen, a suburb of Iquitos, he had already cut the vine into small segments, smashed them with his hammer (so the boiling water could reach into all the various crevices of the vine), and brought water to a boil. He had been smoking mapacho tobacco and singing icaros over the smashed vines when he looked up and saw me there with a large bag of chacruna. He came over to me, reached into the bag, and pulled out a handful, saying very seriously, "Legitimo?"

"Si, Don Juan." And I flipped a leaf over onto its back side and pointed out the tiny darts protruding from the spine. "Legitimo."

Very few of the various mestizo curanderos, who are city dwellers and into the "cash and carry" barter system, actually have their own gardens of ayahuasca vines, and I only encountered two who actually maintained a chacruna bush. What became apparent to me in the numerous rituals with the various healers I experienced was one overriding fact: ayahuasca alone cannot move you through time and space; it requires enough chacruna (*Psychotria viridis*). I did see many different spirits coming into these rituals, but unless I cooked my own medicine, using at least fifty leaves of chacruna or ten leaves of the preferred chaliponga (*Diplopterys cabrerana*) per dose, I never reached the plateau of a full-on entheogenic state. Even when purchasing and cooking my own medicine, I am never guaranteed of its quality because the plants are always varying in percentages of DMT, as they all are coming from different growing conditions and may not have been picked at the proper time of day to insure a higher alkaloid value. The soil in the Peruvian rain forest is mostly sand and clay with two inches of topsoil at most; the lack of nutrients likely produces a lower alkaloid value. The alkaloid content is also highest when the leaves are harvested while they are still moist, before the sun has evaporated the moisture off.

The mestizo curanderos usually have to purchase chacruna from the market or from someone who maintains this bush. This portion of the formula is the most expensive and the most difficult to come by. Because their patients usually don't pay them very well, these curanderos have become accustomed to purchasing only very small amounts of chacruna to cook with their ayahuasca vine. The herbalists in the market normally purchase chacruna from others who grow it in their *chacras,* or private gardens, and have no knowledge of the correct harvesting times. Six soles (two dollars) will get them a small bag containing about sixty leaves. With this, they cook a liter of medicine, or enough to serve twelve people. The correct amount of chacruna per entheogenic dose is, more or less, fifty leaves, depending on the percentage of the alkaloid contained in the leaves. The mestizo curanderos have been cooking their ayahuasca with such a small portion of leaf for such a long period of time they actually believe their formula to be correct. Most likely they never knew the formula, as they were taught by other older curanderos who, out of economic necessity, cooked with very little leaf.

I lightly pounded the chacruna leaves with a mallet for better extraction, then placed approximately half a kilo of the fresh leaves into the ceramic-coated pot. Don Juan was one of the luckier curanderos in the jungle; he had been gifted the cooking pot by a Canadian patron. Normally the pots are aluminum. Don Juan puffed his mapacho cigarette and blew the smoke into the pot, protecting the energies we had given to this medicine and driving away any negative energy that may have been able to conceal itself within its confines. He placed his usual three leaves of datura into the mix and then slowly added the vine and leaves, singing icaros to bless the medicine to give us vision. He cooked all day, pouring the essence into another container each time the water boiled down, leaving only two or three inches in the pot. He repeated this process two more times, saving the essence each time, until only a golden-brown liquid remained. He pulled some of the wood from the fire and slowly began cooking down this essence with less heat. Another hour rumbling on a slow boil and our medicine was complete. We took a short nap, and at nine in the evening we entered the large ritual hut we had recently built beside his home.

That evening, we drank the medicine, hoping to divine a cure for Leonore. As the ceremony began Don Juan asked me to go into a trance and call the spiritual body of his wife before me. I had never attempted this so I followed his instructions with as much focus as possible. Deeply under the influence of the medicine, I called forth a vision of Leonore, concentrating intensely on nothing but seeing her. Just over an hour had passed, and finally I had her form before me. Whether this was simply creative visualization or I actually had succeeded in bringing her spirit there in front of me, I wasn't sure. But I could see Leonore lying in her bed under the mosquito net, asleep, sweating. I looked for her left arm and then to the open wound on her wrist. Don Juan asked me if I could see his wife and I responded "si," without losing visual contact with her image.

"What is it?" he asked. At that instant I knew, as if the word had been planted in my mind. "An insect, maestro."

"Si, Alan," he said, "but how do you cure it?" His voice was fraught with emotion and frustration, as he had been asking me to determine what the remedy for her was and wasn't interested in how it came about. Curanderos have a difficult time seeing and treating members of their own family and generally call on other curanderos to divine for them. I was embarrassed and felt worthless, although I was stunned that the cause of her illness had so quickly issued forth from my thoughts. In that very instant, as I started to apologize for not having given him what he needed, the word "salt" came out of my mouth of its own volition. I hadn't put it there. Indeed, I had not even attempted to divine a remedy at all.

"Salt?" he asked. "How?"

And then I knew. It was clear. "Two spoonfuls of salt in your hand and just a little water to make a paste. Put this directly into the open wound, cover it with your palm, and hold it there for a few minutes."

I had no idea what I was saying or where this cure had come from, but Don Juan understood, sighed in relief, thanked me, and said he would do this at first light.

I was nervous. What had happened here? I explained to Don Juan that I was confused; that this word *salt* had issued from my mouth without my having formed any sort of logical deductions. I pleaded with him not to do this, as placing salt into an open wound would be incredibly painful and, again, I was at a loss to explain where this had come from.

"Alan, this is curanderismo. This is the method of healing. Don't worry."

At first light I hurried into Iquitos to make one last visit to the military doctors. I pleaded with him to wait until I returned, as placing salt in an open wound would be incredibly painful, and I was at a complete loss as to how this word popped out of my mouth. Again, the doctors were of no help, and I returned to the shack to see Don Juan standing in his yard with a cocky grin on his face. I told him the doctors were as confused as I was. He just stood there, smiling at me. It was obvious what he had done.

"You did it, didn't you?" I said.

"Sí."

He had made the salt paste, placing it directly into the wound, and held it there. After a few minutes he removed his hand and a geyser gushed out a pure white creamy fluid, then a liquid watery substance. It was finished. One month later, you could not even see that Leonore had ever been bitten.

Don Juan was forever grateful to me for this healing. After working with him for two years, he slowly became my friend instead of my teacher. He helped me to realize that we are our own teachers. He was my initial guide through the beautifully strange path of the ayahuasquero, until I was able to realize where the soul of this healing came from: it was inside me, just waiting to be activated. Don Juan helped me gain the confidence that has allowed me to continue believing in these strange yet miraculous events that so quickly invaded my soul. He kept me from venturing down a path that could have easily become an endless maze void of soul. I will forever be thankful to him for this.

Two weeks after the ceremony where I had "seen" what had produced Leonore's illness, I walked outside the healing shed during a ceremony to relieve myself, passing my dog, Buddha, on the way. I had gotten him four months after arriving at Don Juan's home, and he had since become the "ayahuasca dog," always waiting outside during ceremony for all the vomiteers to pay their dues. He was our voluntary cleanup crew. One time, I saw him outside lapping it all up, and an hour later

I went to look into his eyes only to see that he was obviously under the influence. Sometimes he would start barking while we were inside the shed conducting ceremony, and I would go outside to see what was causing him to become so agitated, but there was never anything there. It seemed he must have been barking at spirits. Hopefully, I thought, he has learned to discriminate between those that are helpful and those that are harmful.

Buddha had acquired a strange problem with his hair. It began to fall out just under his eyes, and Don Juan told me that I had better take a look at him because the same thing happened to his dog, Volcan, eventually killing him. I looked him over and it didn't seem so bad, but as the days went by it continued and spread, and soon the hair loss got to the point that his upper cheeks were exposed. I thought about taking Buddha to the vet to get a standard remedy for him, but this time, when I glanced at him while under the influence of ayahuasca to see how much of the medicine he had ingested, our eyes met and I suddenly knew how to heal him. It was a strange feeling, similar to my Leonore experience. I leaned down toward him, wiping my fingers to my mouth to collect my saliva, and smeared it over the infected parts below both of his eyes. He seemed to know what I was doing and even held himself still for the treatment. For several days afterward I continued the same treatment, and over a period of three weeks I watched his hair grow back. *Amazing, isn't it?* I thought to myself. By then I had stopped asking myself *Why?* or *How?* because in truth there was no logical explanation. It just was.

THE SPIRIT WORLD

Spirits and the energy of the life force are around us all the time. The Sacred Power Plants such as ayahuasca, San Pedro, peyote, and mushrooms give us sight, allowing us access to spiritual dimensions by removing our ego. Perhaps it changes the vibrational pattern of light entering the retina—I don't know, but for me, this isn't the point. For me, the point is that a spiritual world exists side by side with our ego's waking reality. The spirits come to the curandero, called up by the various icaros he sings. The curandero's ability to master the various shamanic plant diets necessary to learn the path gives him the power to call many types of spirits to counter the many different maladies that exist. The spirits come and imbue the curandero with their power to heal, whether it be physical, psychological, or spiritual. It does not make any difference in which realm the illness resides, they come. These supernatural forces work with and through the curandero, healing the sick in what could best be described as a miraculous way, as these healings are often inexplicable by natural laws as we know them.

Curanderismo is about activating what is known as "the healer within," freeing blocked energy patterns and strengthening the immune system. It is about merging the knowledge of the present with the practices of the past. Medicine is an enabler, allowing the body to heal, but it is the life force that resides within the body that actually does the healing. Medicines may kick off the body's own doctor a little sooner simply because we've been trained to believe in this. It's a conditioned response that our mind will readily accept; in turn it delivers this message to the body that the healing can now begin because we've taken the "medicine." That is why placebos can work. We need to go back to the natural healing methods of the past, when we weren't so dependent on artificial outside forces to make us well. We need an updated belief system that is primarily composed of the traditional healing methods of the past, but combined with the modern New Age healing philosophies of the present. The healer within needs to be understood and activated. This can only happen if the belief system is activated.

The most effective medicine is the medicine we can fabricate inside our own bodies. To get to that it is essential that we contact our own internal doctor. It is here that the ability to cure ourselves resides, for our bodies will actually manifest whatever is necessary to effect a cure. Therefore, we must cultivate the method to activate this healer within. This is made much easier by the ingestion of Sacred Power Plants. Not only do they free the mind, in so doing they allow the possibilities of the healing powers of curanderismo to exist. There exists inside each of us this curandero, the ultimate healer. The key is getting past all the programming by our educational, religious, and social systems, which have molded our modern reality. The modern healer must access what is useful within the allopathic system of medicine, along with the principles of curanderismo. We must work with the concept of the healer within, and also its connection to the spiritual planes of existence. We must recognize that what is sacred and divine exists within us. We are each God. When we leave this physical body we most definitely continue in spirit form. What we make of this very short time in the phenomenal world remains with us after the death of the physical. It is through the use of Sacred Power Plants that these concepts are more easily perceived and assimilated. Once we have activated the Divine, the healer within, we begin to cure ourselves and, in some instances, we may then begin to assist in healing others.

When I speak of the spirit world I refer to those subtle energies continually present but normally just outside our everyday perceptions. We call these energies *spirits*. With the aid of the Sacred Power Plants and a true love for and from them, it is possible to access the spirit world and the spirit doctors that reside there.

Let me be clear: By the use of the word *spirits,* I am not referring to those wispy, translucent forms so often depicted in popular culture. I am not trying to find a way to say that we, as imperfect humans, perceive subtle energies and intellectually alter these into the form of a spirit because we lack the necessary brain capacity to comprehend the energy as it is. Quite simply, spirits were at one time corporeal. They either died, leaving their bodies, or perhaps found that magical, multi-dimensional doorway and walked into another plane of existence (most likely guided by a curandero). They are usually fully clothed, have no odor, and contrary to intellectual opinions, they hear us, speak to us, and we communicate with them. Many speak only the language they died with. Others, more powerful and perhaps more advanced, speak whatever language you need to hear so that you may understand their message. And yes, they do walk through walls. Some may also desire to use your body. In most instances this is not to be allowed, as they can sometimes be difficult to remove. This is the reason for maintaining conscious energy while under the influence of a Sacred Power Plant. This is why you shouldn't fall asleep during any ritual. This is also why you should always sit up when you are taking an entheogenic plant, for just by virtue of sitting up you are maintaining the minimal amount of energy necessary to prevent unwanted energies from possessing you. There are also times that because of the possibility of your spirit leaving your physical body, and in doing so it would appear that the physical body is asleep, you could vomit. If the curandero is not aware of this purging taking place you could be in danger of choking, just like someone who has passed out from drinking too much alcohol.

From time to time other-dimensional energies, both malicious as well as benevolent, find their way into the rituals as well as into your dreams. One month after my initiation as an ayahuasquero, Don Juan and I performed a ritual to determine the reason for a baby's listlessness. He worked on the various possibilities the entire night, questioning the parents thoroughly about their love life and economic situation, but ultimately basing his diagnosis of *susto,* soul fright, on the weak and erratic pulse of the baby. He determined that he must go and visit the house to exorcise the energies present there.

Following the ayahuasca ceremony I retired under my mosquito net to sleep. The dreams you have after a ritual are usually more telling than when in your ordinary sleeping state because your mind is relaxed, in a quiet, meditative state. The ego is out of the way. In this dream a horrible giant in an armored suit was chasing me. The terrain was barren so there was no place I could find to hide. Running, I quickly discovered, was of no use, as this monster was just too quick. When this ugly armored beast approached me for the kill, I was at the point of complete desperation and exhaustion, almost beyond hope. Just then I turned away from it and saw a small elflike person standing just a few feet away from me and presenting me with a beautiful, brightly gleaming stainless steel sword. It was unadorned of precious stones. I felt such exhilaration at that moment because I knew that this sword had magical properties. In one fluid motion I drew it from its scabbard and pivoted around, slicing this shiny blade through the air and decapitating my nemesis. The head bounced off its armored chest and rolled onto the ground. It was finished, I thought. But the beast was still alive and lurching around blindly for its head. I ended it by slicing the head into many pieces. Then I awoke. That morning, while having my post-ayahuasca glass of water with lemon juice and crushed garlic, which is a great liver cleanse, I told Don Juan about my dream.

"Alan," he told me, "you have been presented with a very powerful and dangerous gift."

"Powerful and dangerous? Please explain this to me."

"This gift comes to you from the spiritual plane and will forever be yours to use as you wish. Right now you have been apprenticing for only a short period and it remains to be seen what you will ultimately become—a curandero or a brujo. That's why this sword is dangerous. Yes, you now have a weapon to be used in any way you desire. However, if you ever use this sword for destruction, whatever powers you now have or are yet to receive as a healer will have been compromised. You may carry your weapon with you when you enter the magic of the ayahuasca if you like, or you may simply take note of it and see that it is there from time to time. But you may not use it in destructive ways to bring power to yourself. Its manner of protection for you is in its presence only, that those brujos who might wish to harm you should see it there with you in the spiritual planes and fear to attack you. I remind you again, you should not use it as a weapon. This is your first gift, and many are to follow. If you remain on this path, hopefully you will one day be given a jeweled crown. When this happens I will tell you of its significance."

While this explanation was quite beautiful, I was left with the thought that perhaps I had already compromised myself, having used the sword in my dream. Was I now, unbeknownst to me, on a darker path because of this? Or was the dream a method of gifting me with the sword and demonstrating its power?

Six days later we held another healing ritual, and several poor mestizos came for cures. Sitting on the right-hand side of Don Juan, the position held for apprentices, I began feeling the effects of the medicine within forty minutes. As I went deeper under its influence, I haphazardly glanced over to my left and there it was: my sword, hovering there.

The Sacred Power Plants open your third eye, allowing you to see, but the spirits encountered are not always there for healing. Some come simply out of curiosity, or perhaps they're just bored. In fact, the predominant spirits engaged will not be those called via icaros for healing. I call them wandering spirits, and very often they present themselves in the rituals. At times they can be a nuisance, as I'm a gringo and this keeps them lingering around to watch a fair-haired stranger. If they interfere with my concentration I usually warn them first, then I tell them to leave if they persist. They seem to be neutral spirits, without power. There are others that you may question about various illnesses, however, and their answers are enlightening. These spirits are called via the icaros. I have had much more success calling in these healing spirits when I give them notice that they will be needed. In difficult healing situations I will begin by asking for their presence a week before the healing is to take place. It would seem that they, too, have a life of their own, and to expect that they would instantly appear each time I perform an ayahuasca ritual would be rather presumptuous on my part. And then there are those spirits that come uninvited to the rituals, hoping to cause harm. These can be dangerous. They may even present themselves in the guise of what our mind might perceive as spirits within the energies of the Light. They may use our misperceptions against us by showing up in elegantly flowing white robes, asking us how they may be of service. How can you tell when you are being tricked? Any spirit that will perform something for you that is unethical or immoral is evil. In the shamanistic field of vision, there is good, and most certainly there is evil. They exist in the spiritual plane just as they exist here, in this physical reality.

One month after arriving in Iquitos, Peru, following my canoe trip down the Putumayo, I met a gringo who had been studying curanderismo upriver, near Pucallpa, Peru, with Don Benito and Guillermo Arevalo, two very powerful tribal Shipibo-Conibo curanderos. This gringo was handsome and charming and had a command of the Spanish language and money—all the ingredients needed to bed just about any young, indigent Peruvian lady he desired. And he had been doing just that. Because of this, however, he had also developed a reputation as a womanizer, and to their credit many of the beautiful young Peruvian women would have nothing to do with him. This, of course, only increased his desire for them. During the ayahuasca rituals with his maestros, spirits began coming to him, asking how they could be of service.

"Well, there's this young Peruvian virgin that I'd like to have, but she'll have nothing to do with me," he told the spirit.

"What is her name?" questioned the spirit.

The gringo gave the name, and the spirit told him, "Don't worry. I will arrange this. The next time you encounter this girl she will respond positively to your advances. However, there is something you must do for me in return."

When these spirits first came to him this man thought nothing of it and played along. When the outcome came about as promised, he completely accepted the fact of it. Even at this point he did not go to his maestro for consultation. He had proverbially "sold out," and now he was frightened.

The gringo relating this story refused to tell me what he had done in return for the spirits, and he was full of guilt, embarrassed that he had successfully gone through with the exercise more than once. Now he was frightened of ever drinking ayahuasca again. Finally, after several instances of this during ayahuasca rituals, he told his maestros about it. They were shocked—not only that he had not come to them earlier, but that he had followed through with his end of the bargain with the spirits. He left Pucallpa for Iquitos for this reason, hoping that the evil wouldn't follow or find him.

DIET

There are specific diets for each of the Sacred Power Plants as well as diets for the different "doctors," the term used to describe the spirits of the trees that provide the plant medicine. Depending on which curandero you are working with, the diet will vary. Typically I have found the mestizo curanderos have developed an easier diet for ayahuasca because they have chosen to live in and around the city. In contrast, the diet of the traditional indigenous curanderos is much more demanding; they require much time in solitude and enforce a stricter dietary regime, which is difficult, if not out of the question, for city dwellers. Some of the mestizo curanderos do leave the city from time to time, specifically to diet alone in the jungle. You are usually required to maintain a diet of no salt, sugar, oil, or sex all day before the ceremony and until noon the day after. If you want to learn from the ayahuasca and chacruna (or any other sacred plant that has been added to the ayahuasca medicine), you must diet for a minimum of a week, following the same prescription of no salt, oil, sugar, or sex.

The curanderos I have worked with have all stated that it is dangerous to break the diet, as upon taking the medicine your skin will erupt in red splotches, telling you that the medicine you have in your system has turned against you, red splotches being an outer manifestation of more serious internal damage. However, in my many years of working with curanderos, I have, from time to time, purposefully broken the diet every way possible and have still seen no ill effect. I did this intentionally to ferret out fact from fiction. There were no red splotches, and I didn't get sick.

I have also questioned various curanderos about the requirement of abstaining from sex, and I get no clear answer. I have asked whether this pertains specifically to sex with a partner or if this also includes masturbation. The answers I have received are that you should not "stir" this chakra in any manner, which rules out even exciting this chakra center. Another answer I once received was that it was okay to have sex or excite the sexual chakra as long as you don't orgasm, the theory being that with an orgasm you have nothing to "channel up" when you drink and then purge the medicine.

I must state that although I haven't experienced any negative side effects of breaking the diet, whether it concerns food or sex, I have heard stories from other apprentices who have done so and who have experienced negative consequences as a result. One man had been dieting a very powerful master plant quite strictly for almost a year when he broke his diet with sex. A week later he found himself suffering from a near psychotic breakdown, hallucinating and hearing voices in his head. This is just one story I have heard, and it is very possible that there are others. What I do know, however, is that when you follow the required diet, the spirit world is more accessible. Could it be that salt, sugar, and oil are the ingredients that weigh us down, that separate us from the spirit world? That perhaps these are even venoms to the spirits, such that when they recognize our forms laden with these ingredients they are literally repelled? It has also been my experience that the spirits come more readily after purging either by vomiting or releasing of the bowels.

It was once suggested to me that the diet came about because the curanderos wanted people to respect the spirit of the medicine, participating in the restrictions of the diet and enduring the sacrifice involved in order to show their respect. Hundreds of years ago the most valued items would have been salt, sugar, oil, and sex. I find this an interesting theory, and obviously the psychological state attained from such a sacrifice could not help but produce a beneficial outcome.

Regardless, I have noticed that strictly following the diet is directly related to accessing the spiritual realm. It is my opinion that salt, sugar, and oil work as poisons, and that purging ourselves of these poisons helps us purify our bodies and minds, which in turn helps us become more open and aware of the subtle energies that exist in the world all around us, so that we can perceive and communicate with the entities in the spirit world with much more ease and grace. I also believe that the restriction of sex has come about because this is one of the energies that the spiritual body has had to do without. The more sexual energy you possess, the more likely the spirits will come nearer to and even into you. They desire the sensation, long for it, and this is the closest they can come to it. As a healer once told me, long ago shamans would observe the children in the village in order to determine which ones had more sexual energy. Many times this child would be chosen to continue the shamanic healing lineage.

Sometimes a plant that has been added to the basic drink of ayahuasca requires an even more strict and time-consuming diet. The possibility of learning another plant comes only after you have established a strong relationship with the ayahuasca medicine. You may then add the plant you wish to learn to the basic ayahuasca potion as it is cooking. When you drink the resulting medicine, you can feel in your body where the additive plant goes or, put another way, where it has chosen to do its work, thus enabling you to use it for remedies involving that particular portion of the body.

MY INITIATION

After studying with Don Juan for a year and a half, he decided it was time to present me with my initiation as a curandero. At the time I really didn't understand the significance of this. He explained that the ceremony and the medicines would be under my control. I would be entirely responsible for procuring the vine, chacruna, and datura, and for blessing the plants with the appropriate icaros, cooking the medicine, and determining the dosage for each person. To undergo this initiation I had to strictly follow the required diet: no salt, no sugar, no oils, and abstinence from sex. This wouldn't be that difficult for me as I hadn't added salt or sugar to my food for over twenty years. Oil was a rarity also, so I wouldn't miss this. And sex? I usually found this to be the most difficult, but as this was part of the standard diet for learning ayahuasca anyway I had been somewhat maintaining this regimen since I began my studies, although not always in the strictest sense. I followed this diet for thirty days, and we prepared for the evening of my initiation.

I chopped the vine Don Juan himself had planted several years ago on the small plot of land behind his house, and I blessed the mapacho cigarettes used to *soplar,* blow on, the vine and the ayahuasca as it was cooking. I sang the icaros he used when he cut his vine, hoping that although they were songs taught to me by Don Juan there would be some power within them for me as well. As I pounded the vine in preparation for its cooking, I also sang the icaro Don Juan had suggested, giving it a blessing that the energies released would be of the Light. Don Juan had explained, "This cooking is a very important event in the life of a curandero. It is time to determine what sort of strength you will have as a healer. The stronger the medicine, the more powerful will be the curandero."

As I put the ayahuasca vine, chacruna, and datura into the pot, I prayed for the possibility of activating a strong medicine and that the spirits of the plants would come through. The anticipation of the medicine's effects for this night was constantly on my mind. If I cooked all day and we drank with little effect, I would feel my studies had been in vain. But I had added what I had thought to be the correct amount of chacruna to an amount of ayahuasca vine needed to make ten doses. I had sung the icaros with the correct intent, from my soul, I believed. And even as I continued to stir the pot and hum various icaros, I maintained a state of mind conducive to a beautiful and powerful experience upon drinking the brew. I invited two friends in Iquitos to join me, as this was a special night and I had a very positive feeling that the ayahuasca was going to be as I wanted. This was the first ritual in which I would be in charge. Everyone knew it, and all were hoping it would be a success.

Don Juan and I entered the ritual with small white cloths on top of our heads. We seldom use these, but this night there was only a sliver of moon. The white cloths help the spirits called to understand whom they would be working with. Initially, I sat on Don Juan's right-hand side, the space reserved for me, the apprentice. Although the ritual was under my control, it was still Don Juan who held the position of ultimate authority. I handed a cup of ayahuasca to each person, determining what quantity to pour. This is mostly an intuitive process, watching closely as each person rises from his or her chair and walks up before me. I also use the body weight factor to determine the dose, as this plays an important role in the effects of the ayahuasca. In general, the more a person weighs, the larger the dose. There are those, however, that have a type of spirit that is much more affected by the medicine. All of these factors must be taken into account, but as I said, the intuitive process holds the most weight.

My friends Jim and Marilyn, who were visitors to the country, were the last two to drink. Don Juan and I had previously blessed the medicine, and I had sopla'ed the cup with mapacho smoke. I continued blowing smoke under my shirt and into my hands, waving the smoke up onto my face and over my head, another method for giving protection and blessings. I informed the guests the ayahuasca needed to remain in their system a minimum of twenty minutes, and the longer you could avoid throwing up the more the medicine would work its way into your system.

I explained, "When you need to go outside for purging, it would be best to take a mapacho cigarette; regardless of whether you smoke or not, the smoke will act as a veil of protection for you. Evil spirits do not like tobacco smoke. Besides, it's dark, and they make good flashlights when you puff on them. If you have, at any time, questions about things you see, please ask me. If any spirits present themselves to you, don't be afraid. Ask the spirits what their names are and why they are here."

After we began to feel the effects of the ayahuasca, I blew out the candles and began whistling icaros used to enhance the medicine's effects. As I began feeling more comfortable, I sang other icaros, but not those used to call in the doctors for specific healing. I sang the icaros of blessing and good fortune. The ayahuasca began moving from my feet upward through my legs and into my chest. I could feel it cruising through my body, working its way toward my head. As it neared my ears, the rushing sounds became so loud I could hear no other outside sound for perhaps five minutes. When this passed I began to "see."

Don Juan called the invitees to present themselves, one at a time, in front of him for a blessing after returning from purging outside. I watched as each person had a difficult time walking to him. The ayahuasca was quite strong. As he began the blessings I moved across the room to sit near the door, preventing any unwanted spirits from entering our space.

Don Juan sang a specific icaro for each person, sweeping the shacapa over their body and head, "dusting off" their spirit, cleaning their aura, removing negative energies that may have attached themselves there as a result of living in an industrialized First World. He called for Marilyn, but she had difficulty walking over to him because of the strength of the ayahuasca. I rose and helped place her on the small stool in front of him, then returned to my guardian position near the door. While he was singing an icaro for her, a spirit walked through the wall beside him and continued across the room to stand directly in front of me. I looked it over but most of my concentration and my concern was focused on Marilyn. I looked again at the spirit. It was a man about six feet tall wearing a long, dark, charcoal-colored robe, with a curly black beard interlaced with streaks of silver.

The spirit said, "You wanted to talk to me?" in a heavily Jewish accent.

I had not called this spirit; I had not even been thinking about asking questions of a spirit. My focus was on the present and whether the guests were comfortable, as the ayahuasca was stronger than usual. I looked at Marilyn being enchanted by the blessings of Don Juan and then back to this spirit dressed in a long black robe. I then did what I had previously told my friends absolutely not to do: I did not ask for the name or why the spirit had come. I stupidly looked at this uninvited dark image and whispered, "Vaya," go away.

The spirit nodded, then said, "Okay." It turned around and disappeared, walking through the wall on the opposite side of the room. No other spirits appeared to me that evening, and I spent the rest of the night helping those needing assistance as they went outside of the ritual hut for air to purge, or finally, to retire to their tent to sleep. The ayahuasca had been very powerful and the ritual had been a success. I, too, retired to my mattress and mosquito net and fell into a deep, dreamless sleep. In the morning those who had come to drink with us returned to their homes and to the city's hostels and hotels.

I sat with Don Juan drinking our morning glass of water with lemon juice and garlic, our customary beverage following an ayahuasca ritual. It washes your liver and kidneys of any grainy residues left there by the medicine. Nothing else is to be consumed until noon. Not eating before noon was to allow the full medicinal effects of the ayahuasca to take hold in your body, getting the full amount of healing possible from the medicine. As I sat there with Don Juan he asked me how I thought it went last night.

"The ayahuasca was quite strong," I told him, pleased that it was so.

"Did you experience anything unusual?" he asked me.

"No, Don Juan. I saw only one spirit the entire night." I explained how the spirit looked and how it had presented itself to me.

"With a long black beard and streaks of silver?"

"Yes, Don Juan. And a long, dark, charcoal-colored robe."

"Alan! That was the king, the ayahuasca king! He came to you on the night of your initiation and you sent him away?" He was incredulous. "Didn't I tell you how to respond when a spirit presents itself?"

"Yes, Don Juan. Sorry. Do you think he'll ever come back?" I felt like a complete idiot.

"Of course he will!" he assured me, but I didn't feel very secure with that thought.

The following night I decided to drink again in the hope that this spirit hadn't gone too far away. While I knew the concept of time and space was completely out of place in the spirit world, I still felt that the sooner I could drink, the more likely I would have the opportunity to speak with the king.

That night, in a quite clandestine fashion, I sneaked into the ritual hut and drank a large dose of the very same ayahuasca I had prepared for my initiation. I sat there in the center of the room all alone. When

I felt the effects, I started singing not only the icaros I had learned from Don Juan, but also those from my San Pedro maestro. About an hour into the ceremony, Don Juan came out of his house and entered the hut.

"Alan! What are you doing in here?" He wasn't happy.

"No problem, Don Juan. I'm drinking ayahuasca," I told him, calmly.

"Then sing. Sing the entire time to bring only the spirits you want. If you don't, other undesirables will come."

He then began singing his icaros and demanded I sing along with him. I sang maybe five icaros with him. When he felt comfortable I would continue singing, he started to walk out of the room and got a few feet out when he stuck his head back in the door and said, "You remember the woman from Lima who has been staying here with us?"

Don Juan's family had taken in a young woman from Lima. She was a distant cousin, maybe nineteen years old, who had split with her boyfriend and had come here to repair her heart. She was lazy and slept in every morning after spending every evening out on the town, some-where in Iquitos. She didn't help Leonore with the house chores, the laundry, or cooking but just seemed to sleep and eat. What she actu-ally did during the late hours of the night when she was away from the house was anybody's guess. Daily, Don Juan sang specific icaros that her hurt would be healed soon.

"Si, Don Juan."

"Every night she goes out and returns the next day. I want to know where she is. You go and find her."

"But, Don Juan," I protested, "I'm in the middle of a ritual, drink-ing ayahuasca. I can't leave here now."

He gave me his best "you're not as clever as you think you are" face, and said, "No, Alan. I don't want you to physically go and look for her; I want your spirit to find her. Tomorrow you tell me where she was."

"And how am I going to do this?" I asked.

He shot his look at me again. "So, your other maestro hasn't taught you how to fly yet?" He enjoyed kidding me about things I had and had not learned from my "other maestro." As much as possible, I, too, played with him by not mentioning any of the things I had learned. One of the rules of being an apprentice is that you must completely accept and abide by the philosophy of your teacher, regardless of what you believe. Those things gleaned from previous teachers must be shelved until you have finished the apprenticeship with the current maestro. When you are ready to begin your own practice, you may use those things learned from your various teachers as you will, thus developing your own style as you also integrate those concepts that you personally have discovered and that work for you.

Don Juan continued, "Listen to me. Place the name of the woman on your forehead. Think of nothing else, and go!" He told me, then repeated, "Think of nothing else, and go."

"Gracias, Don Juan." And he left again.

My mind raced. Was this possible? Was this the way to fly? Why hadn't he explained this sooner? As often as I have discovered myself zooming out through space seemingly out of control, I realized I had never simply asked him if there was a rhyme or reason to it. Now he had given me something concrete, as strange as it sounds using *concrete* in this context. I was excited. I sat down in the chair and did as he said. I knew her complete name and placed it into my thoughts, on the very center of my forehead. I found I could maintain this only a minute or so and my mind began wandering. It would come back after wandering off to many other things and I had to begin again. Each time I began anew, I held it longer. Finally, after doing this for what seemed a hundred times, I found myself quite suddenly in the air and moving over the ground at a tremendous speed.

I saw from above the treetops down to the Plaza 28th of July, which was three miles away from Don Juan's ritual hut. I could see the crowds of people and the tiles that made up the walkways. I was hovering above all of this. I didn't get excited; I just looked around, somehow knowing that this, of all the many places this woman could be in Iquitos, was the location I was seeking. I can't tell you with complete certainty exactly what sort of bird or insect it was that I was traveling with, but on looking back I think it must have been a hummingbird or a dragonfly because of the manner in which I was moving, the ability I had to simply hang in midair, and the way I seemed to be wafting back and forth with the breeze. I was looking down into this crowd when a man and a woman turned and walked directly toward me, seemingly presenting themselves. I realized I couldn't actually be seen.

They walked over to be just underneath me. Controlling my excitement that this must be who I had asked to see, I first looked down at the shoes of the woman and man, then the tear in the knee of the blue jeans on the man, to the skirt on the woman. I knew that as soon as I saw her face I wouldn't be able to maintain my calm, so I continued slowly up her body until I reached her face. When I saw her face and realized it was she, my exhilaration was so high it jolted me back into my body in less than an instant. I couldn't believe it! It was real! You not only could leave your body, but it seemed you could even control when and where it happened and possibly even for how long you could stay out.

I was too excited by this discovery to get anything else accomplished for the next hour, so I crawled into my bed to sleep. I couldn't wait to tell Don Juan. I slept through the morning and rose around 11:00 a.m., drank my lemon juice and garlic water, and sat down with Don Juan and his family at noon for lunch.

"Don Juan, I saw her last night!"

He looked up from his bowl of soup. "And?"

"She was at the Plaza 28th of July. She was with a man who had a tear in the knee of his jeans. They weren't touching. It seemed more that they were just friends."

He just shrugged his shoulders and continued eating. About half an hour later, the young woman arrived and sat down to eat. I remember so clearly Don Juan asking her, "Where did you go last night?"

"Plaza 28th of July. I met a friend there."

I didn't even look up from my soup.

There's such magic here, in the jungle. So many things to understand, so many rules to break. And this is only the beginning. The way is full of traps, and it only takes one to fall off your path. The "light at the end of the tunnel" comes from maintaining balance in the midst of adversity. I understand that my mission is not in playing with these tools as a child does a new toy, but in using these gifts of the Sacred Power Plants and the ageless tradition of shamanism for healing. It is here that the real magic resides.

I hope to write more of my experiences in the hope that people might understand this phenomenon called curanderismo, that the troubled missionaries I have so often bumped into might finally understand that this type of work has nothing to do with evil, and to help the travelers who so often come down to the Amazon realize that they too have a healer within. It may not be that they are on the path of becoming a curandero, which is fine. It may just be that they need to understand that they can come to the center of things without trying to become "the shaman."

Don Juan once explained to me the essence of this understanding in the beginning of my apprenticeship. He drew a spiral in the dusty clay at our feet with a twig, and with this twig he began by pointing to the perimeter of the spiral, saying, "Alan, this is the beginning of your studies in curanderismo. As we journey together I will guide you around this outside path and into its inner chambers."

As he said this he moved the pointer to the inner swirls of the vortex. He then stuck the pointer into the center of the vortex and said, "This is the heart of curanderismo and the center that you will have to discover on your own. I cannot and will not show you what lies here. It is for you to discover. When you reach this point you will have learned how to heal yourself, and if the spirits desire, you then will begin to heal others. You will become a curandero with your own methods of curing and a particular group of spirits that you will have begun to work with. While the path of self-healing is for everyone, the ability to heal others is not granted to all. Perhaps, when you reach the heart, you will find that you have learned to heal yourself. Perhaps you will see that this is enough. However, if the spirits of the plants are willing, you will then be allowed to heal others. This we will watch and see."

EPILOGUE

After working in curanderismo for four years in Peru and Ecuador, I received a call from my mother in Tennessee. I hadn't spent any time with her during the previous seven years and only occasionally had written of my experiences. She asked me to come home right away.

"What's wrong?" I asked her.

"Can you buy thalidomide down there in Peru?" Thalidomide was the drug prescribed for morning sickness during the 1950s and '60s, which was later found to have been the cause of thousands of babies being born with birth defects. "I saw a documentary on television the other night praising thalidomide for its curative properties against cancer and AIDS," she said.

"Who has cancer?" I nervously asked her.

"I do." She explained that three-quarters of her liver was cancerous, and she needed to have an operation.

I tried to purchase the thalidomide in Peru but was informed that it had been banned there also. I returned to my teacher, Don Juan, described the situation, and asked if we could perform a ritual to divine the cause and treatment of the cancer. The following night we drank ayahuasca and I saw my mother taking medicine to lower her cholesterol, which was clearly the reason for her cancer. A few nights later we drank again and determined that a bottle of uña de gato (*Uncaria tomentosa*) mixed with jergón sacha (*Dracontium loretense*), two quite powerful plants from the jungle that are anticancer, blood purifying, and boosters of the immune system, would be her best medicine. These plants were to be cooked in a water base to extract the alkaloids, as opposed to using aguardiente, a strong alcohol often made from pulque, which would choke her liver. Don Juan suggested she should drink a glass of room-temperature water and the juice of half a lemon first thing in the morning, followed by a small cup of the uña de gato and jergón sacha blend. I had this advice confirmed by other herbalists in the plant market of Iquitos. Feeling comfortable that this was the correct choice, the medicine was prepared, and I flew out of the jungle to Miami, and on to her home in Tennessee.

"Mother, are you taking any medication to lower your cholesterol?" I asked her.

"Yes, I have been taking Mevacor for years now. Why?"

"This Mevacor is the reason for the cancer."

"No, no!" she insisted. "This medicine is okay—I already asked the doctors; it doesn't cause cancer!"

I let it go, but only after she told me that since her diagnosis she hadn't been taking it anymore. She accepted the medicine I brought her, and every morning for three weeks prior to her operation she drank a glass of water with lemon juice followed by the uña de gato and jergón sacha tea.

When my mother entered the hospital for her scheduled surgery to remove the cancerous portion of her liver, the surgeon, who it just so happened was from Ecuador, advised us that she might not make it through the operation. I had done some research on this type of cancer, hepatocellular, discovering that the possibility of surviving even past one year was quite slim. The liver is amazing in that it is the only organ we have that can actually regenerate itself, but when such a large portion is cut away the shock to the body alone can be enough to kill the person.

After the operation the doctor informed us that the surgery had been successful and that he thought they "got it all." She was in ICU and recovering very well. I asked if he was going to have her diet changed.

"Diet? Why would you want to change her diet? Are you a doctor?"

I explained that a diet of fresh vegetables and fruits with little cooked food would be easier for her system to manage right now as well as provide her with the nutrients she needed. He disagreed. I then told him in one great big mouthful that I had been studying curanderismo in Ecuador and Peru, and that the cholesterol medication she had been taking was the cause of the cancer, and that she had been drinking lemon water followed by the herbal tea every morning for the last three weeks. Then I breathed.

"Mevacor does not cause cancer," he flatly asserted, adding, "I know of uña de gato—it's a folkloric medicine and of little value."

There was no point in arguing with him. I stayed in Tennessee to make sure my mother was recovering well enough and then continued on my speaking tour on the subject of curanderismo, finally returning two months later to Flagstaff, Arizona, which served for a time as my home base in the States. I spent a day researching Mevacor on the Internet and discovered something very interesting: Mevacor lowers cholesterol by combating it in the liver, transmuting it into something else (supposedly more desirable). I telephoned my mother to make sure she had not begun taking the drug again and to re-implant in her mind the necessity of her continuing to drink the uña de gato and jergón sacha tea blend. She agreed. About thirty-five days later, when I was once again in Flagstaff, I received a message to call her.

"Alan, there's something I have to tell you." In those few seconds before she began speaking to me, I considered so many possible dire ramifications of what I imagined she might say next that a sweat broke on my forehead.

"What is it, Mother?"

"Remember the surgeon from Ecuador? He just told me there must have been some error in the radiographs and the sonograms. He apologized, said there was obviously some kind of mistake. When he operated on me, the cancer had shrunk down to a very small size and was completely encapsulated. He can't understand what happened."

"Hmmm . . . but you know what happened, don't you?" I suggested.

"I don't know, Alan. None of this makes any sense. I'm as confused as the doctor is."

"Will you continue to take the medicine I gave you?" I asked.

"Of course I will. By the way, I'm almost out. Can you get me some more?"

With tears streaming down my cheeks, I replied, "Of course. I love you, Mother."

"I love you too, Son."

While studying curanderismo with various maestros, I returned to the United States for a month, stopping in San Francisco to book a return passage with my travel agent. She asked me what shamanism and ayahuasca were all about, and I explained as best I could. She then asked me if it could help her friend who had been diagnosed with an incurable cancer and given only three months to live.

"Absolutely," I told her. "Cancers are one of the diseases that respond best to shamanic healing and ayahuasca. Unfortunately, many people wait until the last gasp to try, making healing all the more difficult." I explained how curanderismo worked, which is a rather unusual subject to speak of in a manner acceptable to those who have no knowledge of it. I myself have been apprenticing for years and have participated in approximately two hundred healing rituals involving either ayahuasca or San Pedro. People come to my maestros for a variety of reasons, and they're coming every day, not simply on the evening of a ritual. However, it is the ceremony with the spirit of the Sacred Power Plant and the curandero that is the most powerful. There is a synergistic magic here. As with the ayahuasca vine requiring the presence of another plant, chacruna, to produce the ayahuasca medicine, so too does the spirit of the medicine require the curandero to effect the cure.

I gave the travel agent my address and returned to the jungle. For the next year I apprenticed with my maestros in Ecuador and Peru and returned to the States, once again stopping to see my travel agent in San Francisco.

"Alan! I have a letter for you," she informed me.

"A letter for me? Who would write me a letter and send it to you?"

"Remember the woman I told you about, my friend with the incurable cancer? I have her letter here. It isn't to you directly, but it's about you and what you told me the last time you were here."

She pulled the letter out of her desk drawer and read it to me. The woman had traveled to Iquitos, Peru, looking for me at the address I had given. She couldn't find me, as I was in Ecuador at the time. She found a guide who took her to a healer, where she participated in an ayahuasca ritual, going into a comalike state for thirty-six hours. Upon awakening she felt extraordinary. Back in the States her doctors performed a battery of tests, finding no signs of cancer. They called it "spontaneous remission"; she called it a miracle. We call it curanderismo.

APPENDIX 1

NO SHORTCUTS

Ayahuasca is the entheogenic purgative preferred by most of the healers in the jungle to alleviate psychological duress, to call the frightened wandering spirit back into the body (soul retrieval), and to divine and transmute physical maladies. La Purga, as many curanderos call it, is the combination of the ayahuasca vine cooked with chacruna; it produces a reaction in the stomach that within forty minutes gives rise to vomiting and/or diarrhea (and in some cases, issuing forth from both ends at the same time). The ultimate bodily effect is one of total cleansing.

The ayahuasca vine (*Banisteriopsis caapi*) contains Beta-carbolines, which deactivate or inhibit an enzyme, monoamine oxidases, or MAO, that occurs naturally in the viscera and the stomach and lower intestines. Once the enzyme has been neutralized, the alkaloid dimethyltryptamine, or DMT, from the admixture of chacruna or chaliponga (*Psychotria viridis* or *Diplopterys cabrerana*) is allowed passage into your system, past your blood-brain barrier.

Instead of taking ayahuasca the traditional way, in which the curandero has brewed it for a lengthy period of time before consuming it, it is possible to extract the necessary alkaloids from the given plants and, once ingested, create an entheogenic effect. The plethora of literature available on the Internet, including the many accessible extraction formulas, makes this a rather simple operation. For example, from the many articles available on the subject, we know that the active alkaloid in the San Pedro cactus is mescaline, and that it resides in only the top eighth of an inch of the skin of the plant. Thus to efficiently produce the entheogen you must discard the remaining part of the plant, as it does not contain any psychoactive alkaloids. Similarly, ayahuasca can be made from an extraction of DMT from a variety of plants (there is even a synthetic DMT) and blended with Syrian rue (*Peganum harmala*) seeds to replace the Beta-carbolines found in the ayahuasca vine.

When I read these kinds of articles, I feel as though I am reading instructions for how to prepare a drug, not a medicine. It is the life force contained in the *entire plant* that activates its healing energies, and it is the manner in which the plant is harvested and prepared and ceremoniously consumed that allows the synergism between us and the plant's spirit and life force energy to effect a cure. When we extract only the alkaloid, we take the plant out of balance. We turn these Sacred Power Plants into something they were never meant to be, and in the majority of instances we create a substance more closely resembling a drug than a true medicine.

It is commonly believed that when you use only the bark of the uña de gato (cat's claw) vine you are very efficiently receiving its medicine. However, in so doing, aren't we also creating a situation whereby our own cellular structure more quickly builds up resistance to the medicine of the whole plant? Addictive drugs are also made by extracting only the potent alkaloids. When the entire plant is used instead, it is more in balance and therefore more likely to keep us in balance. Curanderismo is about healing the *whole* body: spiritually, physically, and emotionally. To accomplish this it is essential that the plants and their specific life forces be allowed to do their work, which cannot happen if only the psychotropic essences are extracted. Certainly you can achieve a visionary experience, cathartic even. As Don Juan has told me many times, "Alan, this is then like a drug. It has no medicinal value."

"Si, Don Juan. It takes the magic away."

APPENDIX 2

THE PRICE OF LEARNING

I hope that for those of you who desire to work with the Sacred Power Plants and enter into the magical realms that exist in the shamanic world, you accept that this comes with a price, which may be difficult to bear: during your journey, not only will you be misled, mistreated, lied to, and manipulated by many of the so-called teachers you will encounter, you will also have to deal with the mental, emotional, and psychological trials and tribulations associated with the shamanic apprenticeship.

Very few curanderos actually have a gift for or were called to do this work. Every one of them will invariably tell you incredible stories of how they used to live with indigenous healers or any number of wild and miraculous stories that they can conjure up to entice you. After all, isn't that what you want to hear? How many preachers or priests have had a "bliss experience"? The truth is, very few. They would all hope for one, whether they tell you this or not. They would all desire to know that the profession they are working in is one of a higher authority, a realm into which they were guided by Divine forces. Rarely is this the case.

It's the same situation with the more or less 4,500 curanderos who practice in the jungles of Loreto, Peru. Many became curanderos because they like the idea. Others do so because there isn't any other work. Cooking ayahuasca isn't a difficult task, and certainly memorizing enough icaros to get you through a ritual is simple enough. And the healing that sometimes comes from their mechanically performing as a curandero, how is this explained? Ayahuasca itself is a very strong medicine, and it alone can provide a cure for many ailments. It is especially good for parasites, one of the most common problems of the rain forest. It's also a very good malaria preventive (after all, malaria is also caused by a parasite). It all comes down to a classic question: How much of the magic is in the medicine and how much is in the curandero? And perhaps more importantly, once your ego is removed, how much of your healing came from your own inner doctor? Would the healing have come had the patient drunk the medicine without the presence of the ayahuasquero?

This is the where I might make a distinction between a curandero-ayahuasquero and a shaman. The shaman is guided to his work. He is on a completely spiritual path of healing. Most ayahuasqueros are mechanics. They have learned their trade as one would learn to become a car mechanic. And this too has a certain power. They do heal, and they are quite knowledgeable about medicinal plants. As a modern medical doctor would notice a symptom and mechanically prescribe a medicine, so too do the curanderos offer plants and herbs for curing. Many of these curanderos are superb psychologists as well; most of the daily problems coming to them involve people with psychological issues, and without such cases they would not be financially able to maintain a practice. They understand also that the majority of physical ailments seen on a daily basis are diet related. And contrary to popular literature very few cases are actually related to evil spells being cast upon the person.

I have great respect for the curanderos I have worked with. Most sincerely desire to heal others, and most are trying to be the most knowledgeable curandero possible. There is now even a licensing school for curanderos in the north of Peru; you too may enroll there.

One final reality check: When I visit with the many curanderos, one fact always emerges: the curandero performs a service and needs to be paid. If there isn't an open verbal exchange of a price for the opportunity to study or drink with them, then one way or another you will find yourself feeling that you have been taken advantage of, that you have been used. And when you can finally get away from it all and are able to sit back and look at what has happened, you will see (or at least I hope that you will see) that your idea of curanderismo and the mystical world of shamanism, that very holy and spiritual place that you so wanted to call home, was not what you had in mind at all.

Many people come to South America with the mistaken impression that this sort of work in a spiritual realm shouldn't be something that one should have to pay for, that the healers should understand you are on a spiritual path and have been guided to them to teach you their methods of curing for nothing, for how can you be charged for such a personal sacrifice? And it is exactly that. It is in the sacrifice of something, whether it be money or a chicken, that allows the teaching to take hold, that enables the healer to heal, the patient to be cured, and the student to be receptive to being given something that they may receive.

I have never outright paid my teachers for anything, as I too had the initial impression that because I knew I was being guided to these apprenticeships I shouldn't have to pay. But I did—it just was never in the direct exchange of money. For example, I built, along with an initial investment made by my friend Gina, a two-story house on my maestro's property over a period of two years. I lived in it, too. Then on December 31, 1995, at 11:55 p.m., I gave the house to him. Had I not, he most likely would have sold it when he caught me out of the country for a couple of months and then moved his family to Brazil. This is simply the way it is in the world of curanderismo, and the sooner you open your eyes and accept it, the quicker you may get down to your real work.

TWO ICAROS FROM DON PEDRO

Here are two icaros given to me from Don Pedro Culqui Vela, of Iquitos, Peru. Don Pedro is a curandero mestizo who also works with ayahuasca, as opposed to a curandero who primarily works with ayahuasca (an ayahuasquero). He occasionally drinks ayahuasca in the small healing room attached to the back of his house, and he gave me permission to publish his address: Bolivar #864. I would suggest that those wishing to visit Don Pedro and join in an ayahuasca ritual go there at least three days ahead of time and pay him upfront so that he can purchase enough chacruna (about five dollars per person). Furthermore, to avoid having to speak about money and having to hear about how difficult it is to survive economically as a curandero, I suggest you pay him for drinking ayahuasca before the ritual begins. A suggested payment is twenty dollars (approximately sixty soles), which is a nice payment for a curandero, especially since you have already given him money to buy the chacruna.

I suggest you follow this advice with any curandero with one caveat: 90 percent of curanderos will thank you for the initial five-dollar payment for the chacruna, accepting the money, and at the same time tell you that it isn't necessary to purchase more chacruna because they are quite efficient at making very powerful ayahuasca. Don't believe them. They will make their typical mestizo ayahuasca, which has, for a liter, not even five dollars' worth of chacruna in it, while pocketing your money. In such a case you should purchase the chacruna yourself and personally place it into the brew being cooked. This is the only assurance you will have that the medicine will contain a sufficient supply of chacruna necessary to produce the desired entheogenic state. I might add that Don Pedro is an exception to this practice.

The first of Don Pedro's icaros is basically untranslatable. It is sung with the right vibrations, using the vocalized sounds I have attempted to transcribe. Some of the lines below include words from the Quechua language mixed with Spanish, which I have attempted to translate.

Sinchi Icaro

Ha na na nai [repeat twice]
Roi ta na na nai
Ta na na nai
Roi espiritista murayari
Espiritista murayari
Sinchi sinchi
Doctorsituy
Ni arnulfo achi de feregros sinchi sinchi
Doctor situy
Ni Curanchiriri cuerpituuy
Ni . . . ni . . . ni . . . ni . . .
Ha . . . na . . . na . . . na . . .
Ta . . . na . . . na . . . noi . . .
Roi cargadito ade [He is coming, carrying many things]
Llegar . . . El legitimo [He's here, the genuine one]
Mediguito [the sweet doctor]
Nunca nunca ya [Never, nevermore]

Ande poder a quebrantar mis [The healing power of
 the icaros cannot be broken]

Icaros . . . Icaros . . . Icaros

The second icaro from Don Pedro is used for calling in the "doctor," the healing spirit of the plant:

El Medico

Dentro la cueva [Inside the cave]

Nasidito [He is born]

Sobre la pena [Under the rock]

Eresidito [He is growing up a little]

De piedra blanca [Of the white rock]

Tu cashimbito [Is your little tobacco pipe]

De tomay penda [Drinking and holding]

Tu tabaquito? [Your little tobacco]

Desde las jaleas [From the honeybees]

A de venir [He will be coming]

Cargadito ade [Carrying many things]

Llegar, El legitimo [He's here, the legitimate one]

Mediquito [The sweet little doctor]

De Chachapoyas [From Chachapoyas]

Ade venir [He's here]

Cargadito ade [Carrying many things]

Llegar . . . El legitimo [He's here . . . the real one]

Mediquito [The dear little doctor]

Nunca nunca ya [Never nevermore]

Nunca nunca ya [Never nevermore]

Ande poder aquebrantar mis [The healing power of
 the icaros cannot be broken]

Icaros . . . Icaros . . . Icaros

GLOSSARY

Aguardiente: A potent alcohol made from the distillation of sugarcane. Medicinal herbs are put into bottles full of aguardiente and shaken several times daily for a couple of weeks in order for the alcohol to extract the medicine from the plants.

Air whistling: Literally carrying the tune of an icaro by whistling without actually bringing forth the notes to full fruition. The melody can still be heard, but it doesn't carry outside of the ritual space. Usually this is done when the cup used to drink the ayahuasca is being sopla'ed, or the mapacho cigarettes to be used during the evening get their blessing. I have also seen an entire evening's icaros performed in this manner in order to hide the ritual from the prying eyes and ears of the outside world, thus keeping the ritual secretive and safe.

Ayahuasca: From the Quechua language, meaning "vine of the dead" or "vine of the soul." *Ayahuasca* is the name used to describe both the medicine made from the combination of the ayahuasca vine (*Banisteriopsis caapi*) and chacruna (*Psychotria viridis*), as well as the name given to the vine itself. It contains harmala and harmaline, collectively known as MAO (monoamine oxidase) inhibitors. It can be found as far north as Panama and is found in the Upper Amazon and throughout the Lower Amazon Basin, where almost every indigenous tribe understands that the vine must be cooked with another plant containing DMT (*N,N*-dimethyl tryptamine) for the medicine to be effective. One of the popular theories among mestizo curanderos is that visitors from outer space or other planets planted the vine here. Because it rarely ever flowers and produces seeds, when you find it growing in the jungle this usually means it has been planted by a healer, is owned by him, and is not to be touched without his permission. I have been lucky enough to see the vine in flower five times since I came to Peru in 1991.

Ayahuasquero: A curandero skilled in the cooking and uses of ayahuasca.

Ayahuasca tourism: There seems to be a movement to convince gringos not to visit with the curanderos of the Amazon of Ecuador, Peru, Brazil, and Bolivia, as doing so "leads inexorably to additional ecological and cultural disruption of affected areas, brings disease to unimmunized Indians, and attracts the wrong kind of attention to ayahuasca."* I have no idea what precisely is being referred to here. I am not aware of any ayahuasca tours that actually take clients so deep into the jungle that they would encounter indigenous people who would otherwise be inaccessible. The indigenous people apparently being referred to in this quote are so far away from civilization as to make it impossible to interfere with their culture or disturb their immune system during a one- or two-week "ayahuasca tourism" program. You simply can't get to them without expeditionary planning. Indeed, the programs I am familiar with in Peru and Ecuador deal primarily with mestizo curanderos and/or tribal cultures that have, as of many years ago, come out of the deep jungle to the commerce areas of the Amazon River and its tributaries. The Indians who have made themselves accessible have done so for economic reasons. Obviously their culture and their immune systems have already been compromised, and they have clearly adjusted. And, fortunately for us, they have brought with them their knowledge of plant medicine. If, from time to time, various ayahuasca tourists visit them, they are more than pleased to share their knowledge. Indeed, they're happy to do so, as their children certainly show no interest in learning it; they're more concerned with "keeping up with the Joneses" by having clean

*Jonathan Ott, *Pharmacotheon: Entheogenic Drugs, Their Plant Sources and History* (Kennewick, Wash.: Natural Products, Co., 1996).

t-shirts and name-brand tennis shoes (the missionaries have made sure of that). I would suggest that those going there bring with them the things cherished the most: pencils and pens, t-shirts (size small and medium), tennis shoes (used ones are fine, size 33 through 37), and shorts. They can be used as trade items for native arts and crafts, or you may gift them.

There are sensitive areas that are accessible, such as the Mayoruna (Matses), but it would require three weeks of boat travel just to get there. Floatplanes are available, but the cost is prohibitive and they hold only a limited number of passengers. I personally believe that expeditions into the far reaches of the jungle, to the tribes refusing acculturation, are disrespectful and dangerous, but I know of no programs that offer this sort of expedition. Perhaps the idea that ayahuasca tourism is a threat to native populations came about because of a report from American author and ethnomycologist Gordon Wasson, who claims to have participated in a *velada,* a mushroom ceremony, with María Sabina, a Mazatec curandera who lived her entire life in a modest dwelling in the Sierra Mazateca of southern Mexico, to which other gringos came without offering sufficient respect for the ceremony, and as a result the spirits stopped speaking to María. However, from the gringos I have encountered who have been in search of ayahuasca, I have to report that the reverse is true: the sacredness of what is involved around curanderismo has very much been maintained and respected by them.

Brujo: The "other side of the coin" of a curandero, they work with black magic. Brujos are healers and they are also in the business of doing danger to people when hired to do so. Usually they have become brujos because they cannot maintain the diets necessary to gain the power inherent in becoming a curandero. In the jungle they prefer to work with the toe plant. Brujos have no scruples and will do virtually anything for money. They can be quite powerful, and once they have done danger to someone it requires a curandero who is stronger than the brujo to remove it.

Chacruna: Local name given to the plant *Psychotria viridis.* Either this plant or chaliponga/huambisa (*Diplopterys cabrerana*) is used as the admixture plant with the ayahuasca vine to make the sacred medicine called ayahuasca. It contains DMT (*N,N*-dimethyltryptamine).

Curandera: A female curandero. In some of the tribal cultures and even within various subgroups of mestizos, curanderas are not apprenticed until after menopause.

Curandero: Luis Eduardo Luna, a very well-respected researcher in mestizo curanderismo, believes it is justified to refer to the various types of curanderos as shamans; I have reservations. Mr. Luna has written by far the most comprehensive reference work on mestizo curanderos: *Vegetalismo: Shamanism among the Mestizo Population of the Peruvian Amazon,* which is currently out of print but deserves to be reprinted by a publisher so that it is accessible to the public. In this work, Luna credits Swedish anthropologist Åke Hultkrantz with this definition of shamanism: "The central idea of shamanism is to establish means of contact with the supernatural world by the ecstatic experience of a professional and inspired intermediary, the shaman. There are thus four important constituents of shamanism: the ideological premise, or the supernatural world and the contacts with it; the shaman as the actor on behalf of a human group; the inspiration granted him by his helping spirits; and the extraordinary, ecstatic experiences of the shaman." I agree that this definition is adequate to cover the mechanics, but it does not address the spiritual qualities necessary within the healer to raise him or her to the level of shaman. I have yet to meet a curandero who has moved beyond monetary and sexual manipulations, not to mention the problems most of them have with their egos. While curanderos understand that any type of adulteration in their life restricts their power, few, if any, can maintain such a lifestyle that would give them the identity of what I perceive to be a true shaman. A shaman, first of all, is a very humble person. A shaman is well beyond petty manipulative games played to extract money or sexual favors. A shaman maintains the powers given him by the gods and the spirits of the plants by maintaining the diet, thoughts, and general conduct of a spiritual person. Nowadays curanderos often refer to themselves as shamans, as they have begun to understand the significance we place on this word, how we put the shaman on a pedestal. My suggestion to those who visit curanderos? If you meet any curandero who refers to himself as a shaman, you should realize that a true shaman would never refer to himself this way and take that into consideration. And know that there are several different types of curanderos: a healer who is a specialist in the uses of ayahuasca is called an *ayahuasquero;* another type of curandero is called a *palero* and is skilled in drinking tree resins. Sometimes ayahuasqueros are jokingly referred to as *sogueros,* as *soga* means "vine" and ayahuasca is made from a vine. Refer to the above referenced work by Luis Eduardo Luna for more detailed information.

Curanderismo: The word comes from the Spanish *curandero,* a person who uses plants as medicine; it pertains to all those things revolving around the healing arts of the curandero.

Datura: The botanical name of this plant is *Brugmansia suaveolens.* Typically no more than three leaves of this plant are added to a curandero's ayahuasca. More than this and you can sense the dryness in your throat. Datura is a dangerously powerful psychotropic that is not to be taken lightly. It is preferred by brujos because they believe that access to the spirit realm is easier through this plant and doesn't require the strict diet necessary for working with other plant teachers.

DMT: *N,N*-dimethyltryptamine is a neurotransmitter found in humans, plants, and animals. The U.S. government has declared it illegal. DMT is the active alkaloid in *Diplopterys cabrerana* (chaliponga) and *Psychotria viridis* (chacruna), the admixture plants used in the ayahuasca brew. The United Nations, in interpreting the Convention on Psychotropic Substances of 1971, which was signed by the United States, has stated that when DMT was declared illegal in the treaty it was referring to DMT in its synthetic form and had nothing to do with DMT occurring naturally in plants or decoctions made from them. However, various governments—those in countries without a traditional use of DMT-containing plants, such as the United States—have stated that their laws override this international treaty and they have made DMT in all its various plant forms illegal.

Doctors: A reference to the spirits of the trees.

Entheogen: "Generating the Divine within." *Entheogen* is now the preferred term to describe what previously has been referred to as "psychotropic" or "psychedelic."

Gringo: From my travels by land down the Amazon I have found that *gringo* refers not only to visiting U.S. citizens but to any stranger visiting any area. It does not have the derogatory significance that it may still have in Mexico.

Harmala and harmaline: MAO inhibitors found in the ayahuasca vine. Monoamine oxidase inhibitors neutralize the naturally occurring MAO in your stomach and intestines. Once your MAO has been shut down, the complete effect of ayahuasca can be felt.

La Purga: Ecuadorian and Peruvian epithet used to denote the ayahuasca drink. In English it means "the purgative."

Mapacho: *Nicotiana rustica,* a richly flavored jungle tobacco grown upriver from Iquitos, Peru. The leaves are rolled into small, ten-inch-long, two-inch-thick sticks after they have been dipped in the local moonshine made from a distillation of sugarcane (i.e., *aguardiente*) to prevent molding.

Mestizo: This is the race that has been created by the mixture of indigenous and Spanish genes.

Sacred Power Plants: Those plants that when ingested produce extasis. They are sacred by virtue of their being entheogenic. They all possess a healing spirit or entity within them that can possibly become your teacher if it chooses to show itself to you.

San Pedro: The psychotropic cactus *Trichocereus pachanoi.* This is perhaps the fastest-growing cactus in the world and has not been declared illegal—yet. It contains mescaline and is a Sacred Power Plant used in the Andes of Ecuador and Peru.

Soplar: In the ayahuasca ritual this refers to the action of breathing in the smoke from sacred tobacco and blowing it over an object or person, the reason being to purify and protect what it has been blown onto. Typically you are sopla'ed with either organic mapacho tobacco smoke or with agua florida. However, these days the agua florida is synthetic and slightly burns the mouth. Best is to make your own using aguardiente or 151 vodka. Put aromatic herbs in the bottle for a couple of weeks and shake often.

Tambo: A thatched-roof, open-walled hut.

Vaya: Spanish for "go away."

Vegetalista: A vegetalista is one who cures using the *vegetals,* or plants, and is usually a curandero who has also mastered one of the tree resins.

ABOUT THE AUTHOR

Alan Shoemaker makes his home in Iquitos, Peru, with his family. He studies mestizo curanderismo and sometimes guides others to the maestros of Ecuador and Peru. He hosts the annual International Amazonian Shamanism Conference (www.vineofthesoul.org), held every July in Iquitos, and heads DragonFly Tours, a travel agency booking interior Peruvian flights for tourists. He also holds Vine of the Soul Intensives in a ceremonial chapel just twenty minutes up the Itaya River from Iquitos (www.facebook.com/groups/vineofthesoulintensives).

Alan Shoemaker can be reached at

alanshoemaker@hotmail.com

INDEX

"Adan Visionario," *pl.1*

agua florida, 23, 50, 134–35

aguardiente, 129

AIDS, xi, 3

air whistling, 129

alkaloids, 1, 90, 120–21

allopathic medicine, 12

animal spirits, 63–64

antibiotics, 44

apprentices, 44–45, 123–25

Arevalo, Guillermo, 100–101

atropine, 43

auras, 23–24

ayahuasca, 129–30

  effects of, 35

  traditional preparation of, 120–22

  See also specific topics

ayahuasca tourism, 130–31

bad energy, 49

balance, 121–22

belief systems, 96

bells, 23

Benito, Don, 100–101

Betacarbolines, 65, 73, 120

biches, 24

bipolar disorder, 73

black magic, 85

bliss experience, 123

boas, 41

brujeria, 85

brujos, 47, 52, 56, 85, 131

Buddha (dog), 93–94

caiman and monkey soup, 83

cancer, 115–19

Capp, Al, 30

Castaneda, Carlos, 53

centering, 79

chacras, 90

chacruna, 73, 89–91, 106, 120, 126–27, 131–32

chaliponga, 43, 90, 120

character traits, 49–50

cigarettes, 82, 107

clairaudience, 30

cleansing, 26–27

clearing, 73–74

cocaine, 2–3

cooking, 105–6, 124

cooking pots, 91

Culqui Vela, Don Pedro, 126–28

curanderos, 132–33
  activating healer within, 95–96
  heart of, 113–14
  price of learning, 123–25
  stereotypes of, 37–38
  use of term, 4

datura, 43, 56, 73, 91, 133

death, symbolic, 34

Debernardi, Anderson, *pl.1–pl.3*

Dickinson, Emily, 24

diets, 44–45, 83, 102–4

Diplopterys cabrerana, 90

Divine, 2, 96

DMT, 73, 90, 120, 121, 133

doctors, 134

dosage, 106–7

Dos Hermanos, 59

Dracontium loretense, 115–16

Drake, Stan, 30

dreams, 97–99

drugs, 121

ego, 13, 14, 98

elementals, 51

El Medico, 128

emotional growth, 49–50

entheogens, 134

ethics, 44

evil, 69, 79, 100

Fatima, Don Jose, 19, 61–64

Fernando, Don, 65–74

flying, 110–13

focus, 53

gardens, 90

Gina, 61–62, 65, 68–73

God, 44, 96

good, 100

Gorman, Peter, ix–xvii, *pl.8*

gringos, 44, 134

guayusa tea, 16, 25–26

habits, 35

Hampjes, Valentin, 6, 11–17,
  49–58, *pl.8*
  background of, 18–20
  vision of orphanage, 21–22

harmala, 73, 134

harmaline, 73, 134

harmonicas, 43–44, 77

healer within, 95–96

healing, 12–13, 83, 85–94, 115–19,
  124–25

healing songs. *See* icaros

healing spirits, 100

Heliconia flowers, *pl.6*

hepatocellular cancer, 116

"holy men," 37–38

Hultkrantz, Åke, 132

hyocyamine, 43

icaros, 19, 35, 47, 75–79, 126–28

illness, 12–13, 85–94

immune system, 3, 12–13

Inchaustegui, Roberto, xi–xii
information, 29
"Iniciacion Shamanica," *pl.2*
initiation, 105–14
internal doctor, 35
intuition, 29
Iquitos, Peru, 33, 34, 47–48, 80

jaguars, 41–42
jergón sacha, 115–16
Jewish spirit, 108–9
Joe (schoolteacher), 4–6

kidney cancer, 57
king, 108–9
Krishna consciousness, 12

La Chorrera, Colombia, 36
languages, 77
La Purga, 134
lashing, 26
Laura, 80–82
learning, price of, 123–25
lemon water, 116
Leonore, 83, 88–89, 91–93, *pl.8*
Light, 76, 79, 100
logging, 66–67
Lord's Prayer, 57
Loreta, Peru, 123–24
Luna, Luis Eduardo, 76, 132

Mabit, Jacques, 2–3
Madann, 54, 55
magic, 29, 122
malaria, 124

manchas, 23–24
mantas, xvi
mapacho cigarettes, 107, 134
Marilyn, 107, 108
Mayoruna, 131
medicine, 95–96
medicine men, 73–74
Mevacor, 116–17
miracles, 29
missionaries, 44, 113, 131
Mohito, 15, 23, 25, 26, 28, 50, 54,
    56–58
money, 125, 126–27
monkey, 83
monoamine oxidases (MAO), 120
Montes, Francisco, xi
Muridunga, 15, 20
mushrooms, 95

negative energies, 76, 79, 97–98,
    100, 108
negro ayahuasca, 73
Nerhu style, 60
New Age, 96
Nostradamus, 22

oil, 102–4
orphanage, 21–22
Osta, Andrew, *pl.4–pl.5*

paleros, 133
palm leaves, 23–24
palo santo, 73–74
parasite medication, 44
parasites, 124

patterns, 35, 49–50
payment, 125, 126–27
Pedro, Don, 126–28
Peganum harmala, 121
Perea, Jorge Pandura, xiii
Perez, Mauro Reategui, *pl.6–pl.7*
perfectionism, 37–38
peyote, 95
phlegm, 25–26
Pio Putumayo, 35–36
placebos, 96
possession, 75–76
posture, 97
psychological programming,
    28–29
psychotic mental states, 75–76
Psychotria viridis. See chacruna
Pucallapa, Peru, 61, 100–101
Puerto Asis, Colombia, 36
purging, 40, 107

quantum physics, 2
Quechua, 76

Requena, 65–66
response patterns, 35, 49–50
ritual, 29, 97–98
Roberto (travel companion), 5
"Russian Fairytale," *pl.5*

Sabina, María, 131
Sachamama Ethnobotanical
    Garden, xi
Sacred Power Plants, 1, 3, 12–13, 134
    dangers of, 75–76

diet and, 44–45
effects of, 35, 49–50
healing and, 95–97
salt, 102–4
"Salvia Ceremony," *pl.4*
San Pedro cactus, 12, 15, 17, 18–27,
    121, 134
Sasha, 31–33, 58
Sasha (woman), 61–62
scopolamine, 43
seguro, 26
sex and sexuality, 42–43, 68, 83,
    102–4, 105
shacapa, 23–24, 50
shamans and shamanism, 1, 2,
    37–38, 124, 132–33
    definition of, 132–33
    gringos as, 44
    rebirth of, 3
Shoemaker, Alan
    animal spirits and, 63–64
    apprenticeship of, 80–94
    breaking through barriers, 28–33
    contact with mother, 115–17
    diet and, 102–4
    Don Fernando and, 65–74
    first ayahuasca experience, 35–46
    Gormon on, x–xvii
    initiation of, 105–14
    pictured, *pl.8*
    on power of icaros, 75–79
    quest of, 4–6
    return to Ecuador, 47–60
    San Pedro experiences, 18–27,
        49–58

in search of a maestro, 34–46
on soul dusting, 23–24
sword dream of, 98–99
synchronicity and, 7–10
Valentin and, 11–17, 49–58
Shoemaker, Albert Thomas, 29–30
short-term memory, 31
Sinchi Icaro, 127–28
Siona curandero, 34–38, 77
sitting, 97
sixth sense, 29
sleep, 97
snakes, 86–88
sogueros, 133
soplar, xiv, 134–35
sorcery, 7–8
soul dusting, 23–24, 50–51
soul fright, 98
soul loss, 75, 120
space preparation, 73–74
Spanish Inquisition, 1
spirit of the plants, 76–77
spirits, 40–41, 56–57, 66–67,
    68–72, 95–101
stinging nettles, 26
sugar, 102–4
sugarcane, 39
susto, 98
sword dream, 98–99
synchronicity, 5–6, 7–10
Syrian rue, 121

Tangoa, Don Juan, 34, 49, 80–94,
    105–14, *pl.8*
telepathy, 29
thalidomide, 115
Thea, 42–43
third eye, 99–100
tobacco juice, 15, 25–26, 50
"Trance Shamanica," *pl.3*
two-headed snake, 86–88

uña de gato, 115–16, 121
Uncaria tomentosa, 115–16

*Vegetalismo: Shamanism among
    the Mestizo Population of the
    Peruvian Amazon,* 76, 132
vegetalista, 135
Vilcambamba, 21
Virgin Mary, 52, 54
visions, 13
vomit, 40, 107

wandering spirits, 99–100, 120
Wasson, Gordon, 131
weight, 106–7
White, Timothy, ix–x
white cloths, 106
white horse story, 25
Willy, 83

Yage Letters, The, x

BOOKS OF RELATED INTEREST

The Ayahuasca Experience
A Sourcebook on the Sacred Vine of Spirits
Edited by Ralph Metzner

Ayahuasca
The Visionary and Healing Powers of the Vine of the Soul
by Joan Parisi Wilcox

The Religion of Ayahuasca
The Teachings of the Church of Santo Daime
by Alex Polari de Alverga

Black Smoke
Healing and Ayahuasca Shamanism in the Amazon
by Margaret De Wys

The Psychotropic Mind
The World according to Ayahuasca, Iboga, and Shamanism
by Jeremy Narby, Jan Kounen, and Vincent Ravalec

Plant Spirit Shamanism
Traditional Techniques for Healing the Soul
by Ross Heaven and Howard G. Charing

Plants of the Gods
Their Sacred, Healing, and Hallucinogenic Powers
by Richard Evans Schultes, Albert Hofmann, and Christian Rätsch

DMT: The Spirit Molecule
A Doctor's Revolutionary Research into the Biology of Near-Death and
Mystical Experiences
by Rick Strassman, M.D.

INNER TRADITIONS • BEAR & COMPANY
P.O. Box 388
Rochester, VT 05767
1-800-246-8648
www.InnerTraditions.com

Or contact your local bookseller